Nursing
Observation

14-12

D0492460

FOUNDATIONS OF NURSING SERIES

WM C. BROWN COMPANY PUBLISHERS

NURSING OBSERVATION, *Virginia B. Byers, Pleasantville, Pennsylvania*

PROMOTING PSYCHOLOGICAL COMFORT, *Gloria M. Francis and Barbara Munjas, Medical College of Virginia*

THE FASCINATION OF PROBLEM SOLVING, *Mae M. Johnson and Mary Lou Chamberlain, Los Angeles Valley College*

COMMUNICATION, *Garland K. Lewis, Catholic University of America*

WORKING WITH OTHERS FOR PATIENT CARE, *Grace Peterson, DePaul University*

TEACHING FUNCTION OF THE NURSING PRACTITIONER, *Margaret L. Pohl, Hunter College*

PROMOTION OF PHYSICAL COMFORT AND SAFETY, *Valentina G. Fischer and Arlene Connolly, Boston University*

Nursing
Observation

Virginia B. Byers
Formerly Assistant Professor of Medical Nursing
University of Pittsburgh
Pittsburgh, Pennsylvania

WM. C. BROWN COMPANY PUBLISHERS, *Dubuque, Iowa*

Nursing today is experiencing new developments in basic knowledge and practices. The appearance of new concepts, along with greater diversification in health care facilities, has created a demand for nurses equipped with the knowledge and abilities to promote health, prevent disease and injury, and care and comfort the helpless and sick.

The **Foundations of Nursing Series** is in response to the need for new educational material in the field. The individual volumes in this Series include the knowledge and skills now being incorporated into modern nursing practices. This Series offers both the student and teacher flexibility of subject matter, as well as authoritative writing in each text area. Although the individual titles are self-contained, collectively they cover the major subjects, as discussed in introductory courses.

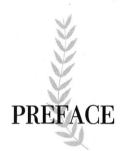

PREFACE

This book is designed for beginning students in nursing and is based upon the premise that the professional nurse must possess certain highly developed skills, one of which is observation. Basic to the development of any skill is knowledge of the facts which support it. In the case of nursing observation, this supporting knowledge is drawn from the vast areas of the natural and social sciences. It consists of an understanding of the structure and function of the human body in health and of the changes that occur as a result of illness.

The purpose of this book is to provide the student with a knowledge of specific observations to be made as she administers nursing care even in the very early stages of her career. Observation of the patient is complicated by the fact that the beginning student is confronted with so many adjustments and challenges in her new role of ministering to the sick. This book is intended to serve, along with the other books in this series, as a text for the first clinical course in nursing, or Fundamentals of Nursing. Individually, it can serve as a useful reference to any nurse in a clinical setting.

An introduction to the role of observation in nursing practice, including the methods of observing and the interpretation and evaluation of observations is basic to the understanding of the importance of more specific observations. A discussion of selected general observations of people provides a background for moving toward the more specific observations of signs and symptoms in the care of the sick. A representative group of frequently performed nursing activities has been selected to illustrate the observations to be made by the nurse as she performs various nursing techniques. The last section is devoted to patient situations which require the nurse to apply her knowledge of nursing theory in order to make significant observations.

Although other basic nursing texts have included discussion related to the skill of observation, it is believed that this is the first book to be devoted entirely to this subject. It is hoped that this book will help the student to become more aware of the specific needs of the patient and that, in conjunction with knowledge gained through other courses, effective approaches to meet those needs can be found.

VIRGINIA B. BYERS

CONTENTS

Chapter _____ 1

The Role of Observation
in Nursing Practice

Patterns of educational preparation of the professional nurse have changed greatly since the days when Florence Nightingale recruited and trained young women to help her in the care of the sick and wounded. Actually, her task was complicated by the fact that the merits of professional nursing had not been established; through her practice, she had to prove that what she was saying was true and necessary. From the days of apprentice-type training, nursing education has evolved into very specialized education. The facilities for learning have been expanded to include the college classroom and the experimental laboratory as well as the clinical laboratory of the hospital.

Methods of teaching have changed drastically, too. With the use of audio-visual materials and systems ranging from simple drawings to the most complex apparatus for closed circuit television production, students are afforded an opportunity to gain a more graphic understanding of what is required of them as professionals in a health field. The availability of reference books, manuals, professional publications, and individual teaching machines have made it possible for the student to assume responsibility for learning through guided but independent study.

Although many changes have been implemented in the area of methods, equipment, and facilities for nursing education, the professional nurse of today must possess many of the same personal characteristics as did her predecessors. These are the personal qualities that cause a person to want to spend her life helping those who are sick. One of these qualities is the attitude of selflessness which enables one to recognize and grant priority to the needs of others. This is an attitude which comes through maturity and self-discipline. Another characteristic is a deep personal commitment to the welfare of others and to the goals of the nursing profession. Still another characteristic is a willingness to assume responsibility for the care of others even when this care requires sacrifice of personal desires and the performance of tasks which seem mundane and aesthetically unappealing.

DEVELOPMENT OF SKILL IN OBSERVATION

In order for the nurse to meet the responsibilities that she has assumed, she will need to develop certain basic skills. One of these skills is observation of the patient. The term observation can be used in various ways ranging from simply seeing an act or object to a perception of what is being seen with an understanding that enables one to make an interpretation or to draw a conclusion. Observation as a nursing skill is not a simple skill which just comes with practice. The word skill suggests a highly developed ability. Thus, skill in observation means that the person making the observation possesses an expertness in the ability to observe. Basic to the development of expertise in observation is a core of knowledge of the natural and social sciences as they relate to the functioning of the human being. The nurse must know what she is looking for and when to expect it as well as what steps to take when she finds it. Skill in observation, then, implies that there is a real perception of the situation being observed.

The main difference between perception and seeing is that perception connotes understanding of what is detected through any of the various senses. This means that the nurse must seek knowledge which enables her to understand what she observes in her patients and to apply this knowledge in all of her nursing experiences. The inclusion of perception as a part of nursing observation does not imply that the nurse makes a medical diagnosis but that she will be able to apply her knowledge to determine whether observations made suggest deviations which should be brought to the attention of the physician or that she will be able to handle the situation without further guidance. The use of good judgment is an essential part of nursing practice.

Skill in observation does not come spontaneously with the mastery of the various academic and clinical courses specified in a curriculum. The development of this skill is a long and arduous process of deliberate consideration of patients and the problems they present. To the novice, only the major aspects of a specific situation will be obvious. With concerted effort, the nurse can apply her basic knowledge to her encounters with patients and can become so skillful in observing patients and their problems that, from a brief encounter, she can identify the problems which require nursing assistance.

Knowledge of the scientific basis for nursing is a requisite if the nurse is to grasp the full meaning of her observations. Traditionally, emphasis has been placed upon the natural and biological sciences in nursing curricula. As a result of research in the social sciences, they, too, have been recognized as having an important place in nursing education. A knowledge of the dynamics of human behavior during a state of good health enables the nurse to recognize and appreciate changes brought about by illness. Illness has an impact upon the patient and his family, and an understanding of this fact enables the nurse to accept them and to minister effectively to all of them. A lack of understanding on the part of the nurse leads to frustration for all concerned. Such frustration interferes with communication, and poor communication stands as an impediment to treatment and progress of the patient.

Before a nurse can help any patient, she must consider what she knows about him, his illness, his strengths and weaknesses, and then make an assessment of those areas of need in which she can be helpful. In essence, this is what is meant when the term nursing diagnosis is used. Nursing diagnosis refers to the decisions that the nurse must make regarding the kind and extent of assistance to be rendered to meet the needs of a patient. As the nurse becomes more skillful in this process, she will know the limits of nursing practice and will request the services of a physician or other member of the health team at the appropriate time. Although an important function of the nurse is to carry out the prescriptions of the physician, there are some functions which she can perform independently. Observation is one of these functions, and it is often the nurse who is the first to detect changes in the condition of a patient. This observation is facilitated by the continuity of nursing care.

Changes in the pattern of hospital stay and methods of treatment of patients have added to the complexity of observation of patients. As the length of hospital stay decreases, the nurse finds herself responsible for more patients who are in the acute phase of illness. The more acutely ill the patient, the greater is his need for constant and scrutinous observation. Thus, the demand for skillful observation is increased. As patients regain sufficient strength to assume responsibility for their physical care, they leave the hospital only to make room for more patients who are acutely ill.

Modern hospital construction demonstrates the importance of observation in the care of the sick through the extensive use of glass walls, observation rooms, and one way mirrors which facilitate the constant observation of patients. The central location of nursing stations enables the nurse to maintain a more constant watch over her patients, especially those whose condition warrants it.

Although the use of some of the newer equipment available for patient care appears to complicate the task of the nurse, it offers great benefit to the patient. For example, the pacemaker makes possible a kind of treatment which can mean the difference between life and death for someone. The various monitoring devices which can be used to observe and record a detailed account of the physiological processes of the patient enable both nurses and physicians to detect significant changes much earlier than would be true if these machines were not available.

In order to use these machines intelligently, there are some things that the nurse must know about the machine itself. No nurse is expected to know all of the details about the operation of machinery of this type, but she must be able to recognize signals emitted by the machine when there is a disturbance in its function so that she will be able to enlist the aid of the engineer who is responsible for its maintenance. When a nurse assumes responsibility for the care of patients whose care involves the use of any of this machinery, she must assume responsibility for learning what to do when emergencies arise. Otherwise, she may find herself in the predicament of a nurse who was called to a patient's room by the ringing of a bell which was located in a pacemaker. When she arrived, she found both the patient and his wife in a very apprehensive state because they knew that the patient's very life depended upon this machine. Neither this nurse nor any other nurse on the unit knew how to make the bell stop ringing without disrupting the function of the machine. Fortunately, in this case, the ringing of the bell proved to be a false alarm, and no harm came to the patient except that his confidence in the nurses in attendance was destroyed.

Another point worthy of mention here is the fact that monitoring devices are not intended to take the place of nurses, but rather they are to enable nurses to elevate the quality of care given. Application of scientific knowledge is essential to the intelligent use of information provided by the machine.

Other types of treatment which intensify the need for skill in observation are treatment with powerful drugs and newer surgical techniques. Improved techniques in the administration of anesthetics and the development of equipment which will perform the functions of such vital organs as the heart, lungs, and kidneys have made possible types of surgery that were unknown in the first half of this century.

Such surgery requires intensive observation and nursing care during an extended period of recovery.

As new drugs are developed through research, they are made available for administration to patients in hospitals. Their release is not made, however, until they are considered safe for general use. The nature of some of these drugs, though they may be life saving, is such that they can produce drastic side effects. These adverse effects may not occur in every patient, but it is the responsibility of the nurse to observe all patients receiving medication so that their well-being can be safeguarded. Such observation requires the nurse to assume responsibility for learning about any drug that she administers.

While the foregoing paragraphs have dealt with developments which have added to the complexity of observation and nursing care, it should be emphasized that changes in many of the nursing techniques have made it possible for nurses to focus their attention upon the real needs of patients. Historically, some nursing procedures such as bathing and making the bed of the bedfast patient have included such ritualistic aspects as measuring the distance between the edge of the draw sheet and the head of the bed. As nurses have come to realize that such time-consuming steps add nothing toward meeting the comfort or any other need of the patient, nursing procedures have been revised. Many other time-consuming tasks have been eliminated from the realm of nursing responsibility through the use of disposable equipment and through better utilization of nonprofessional personnel. Consequently, the time has been made available for the nurse to use her skill in observation and to make use of the data gained as she offers assistance to those whose disability makes it necessary.

METHODS OF OBSERVATION

As has already been established, nursing observations consist of more than cursory notations of obvious deviations in the condition of a patient. Skillful observation employs the use of the various senses of sight, touch, smell, and hearing as guided by the scientific knowledge which comprises the basis for professional nursing. In addition to knowledge of the normal anatomy and physiology of the human body, the nurse must have a working knowledge of changes that occur as a result of disease or injury. Signals or evidence of these changes are commonly called signs and symptoms. The term sign is applied to those changes which are detectable by the observer such as discoloration of the skin, edema, and jaundice. The term symptom is applied to phenomena which are apparent only to the affected person.[1] Examples of symptoms would be pain and itching.

Another means of classifying symptoms is to use the categories of objective and subjective. Objective symptoms are those symptoms which can be observed or measured by another person, while subjective symptoms are those symptoms experienced or felt only by the affected person. Information relating to subjective symptoms must be elicited from the patient through the use of pertinent but nondirective questioning.

When one thinks of the term observation, the first sense to come to mind is sight. Its importance cannot be underestimated. Even when a patient is experiencing the symptom of pain, there may be changes in the facial expression which will serve as the first clue indicating that the patient is uncomfortable. There will be many instances, however, when other senses must be employed, either separately or in conjunction with sight. For example, it is possible for a patient to have a subcutaneous mass which can be detected only through palpation. In addition to its function of serving as a means of observation, touch is an instrument of communication. The attitude of the nurse is conveyed to the patient through touch as the nurse performs such measures as backrubs and offering assistance in walking or changing position. Likewise, the nurse can discern from the patient's touch as he reaches for support something about his attitude.

The sense of smell, though a less obvious method of observing, does enable the nurse to detect problems pertaining to the patient and his environment. In some cases, odors may be the result of poor hygiene. Sometimes, however, odors are related specifically to the patient's medical problem. For example, certain pathologic conditions produce odors which, if not always offensive, may be significant. An example is the characteristic odor of the breath of a person who is suffering from diabetic acidosis. One of the serious aspects of this condition is the high level of acetone contained within the blood. The presence of the acetone is caused by the inability to metabolize fats. As is the case so often, when this physiologic disturbance occurs, the human body automatically attempts to adapt itself so that it can maintain equilibrium or homeostasis. Because improper metabolism is producing a toxic waste which must be excreted, a channel for its excretion must be found. One channel by which it can be excreted is through the respiratory tract, hence, the sweet, fruit-like odor of the breath.

Detection and prompt removal or control of noxious odors is important in the maintenance of a pleasant environment in the hospital.

---

[1]Cyril Mitchell MacBryde, *Signs and Symptoms* (Philadelphia: J. B. Lippincott Company, 1964), page 1.

The use of deodorizing agents along with good ventilation helps to reduce the problems caused by body wastes and volatile agents such as disinfectants. The use of these agents does not preclude the necessity of cleanliness, however. Because of the hazardous nature of fire, especially in a hospital, the nurse should be alert to the presence of smoke so that a safe environment can be maintained.

The sense of hearing is associated primarily with communication, but in nursing, it plays an important role in techniques which require the use of a stethoscope. For example, the nurse must learn to identify the sound of the heart so that she can measure the blood pressure or can obtain an accurate count of the apical pulse. Sometimes, the nurse may find it necessary to use the stethoscope to listen for the quality of respirations or peristalsis. As the nurse listens to the verbal communication of the patient, she must listen in such a way that she hears what he is saying as well as the way in which he says it. The nursing responsibilities related to listening are discussed in more detail in Chapter 4.

TOOLS TO AID IN OBSERVATION

In addition to the direct observations which can be made through the use of the various senses and measuring devices, some other tools which will be helpful in developing skill in observation are check lists and process recording and evaluation of interviews. The main purpose of a check list is to serve as a guide to those characteristics or symptoms presented by a patient. Just as the beginning student finds a list of specific tasks and responsibilities to be helpful in completing an assignment, so the nurse meeting a patient for the first time will find a check list to be helpful in assessing the condition and needs of a patient.

The hospital procedure committee may find it helpful to compile a list of observations to be made as a part of the admission procedure. A detailed example of a check list of observations to be made by the nurse can be found in Beland's *Clinical Nursing: Pathophysiological and Psychosocial Approaches.*[2] This list of specific observations includes physical and psychological aspects. Using such a detailed list as a guide, the individual nurse can construct a list which is adapted to her particular situation.

As the nurse develops proficiency in the observation of overt or obvious signs or symptoms of problems, she will need to keep in mind that covert problems exist also. Covert, or less obvious, problems are

---

[2]Irene L. Beland, *Clinical Nursing: Pathophysiological and Psychosocial Approaches* (New York: The Macmillan Company, 1965), pages 22-30.

often related to psychosocial factors. They may be related specifically
to the illness of the patient, or they may be of a more general nature
arising from difficulty in his personal adjustment to the problems of
everyday living. Whatever the nature of the problem, it is most effectively observed indirectly. As the nurse establishes a relationship of
trust with the patient, he is often able to discuss problems that he
considers too confidential to discuss with strangers, doctors or nurses.
Conversations or interactions occurring coincidentally with nursing care
provide an excellent opportunity for the nurse to listen to the patient.
It should be emphasized that, contrary to the early thinking in nursing,
the nurse does not need to be administering physical care to a patient
to justify the time spent with him listening to a problem.

Because nurse-patient interactions provide an excellent source of
information related to the specific needs of the individual, the nurse
should develop the ability to reflect upon such interactions to evaluate
her effectiveness. A verbatim recording of the conversations will permit
the nurse to review the entire interaction. Since mannerisms, attitudes,
and general behavior reveal considerable information about a person,
any such action should be recorded along with the words spoken. The
questions and comments offered by the nurse should be recorded, also.
This detailed account of a nurse-patient interaction is called a process
recording. In order to evaluate the interaction, it might be helpful to
use a three-column plan, one for the remarks and actions of the patient,
one for the remarks and actions of the nurse, and the third for the
evaluation by the nurse. An example of this type of evaluation of an
interview or interaction is presented by Bermosk and Mordan in their
book, *Interviewing in Nursing.*[3]

Although this practice of evaluation can be tedious and time consuming, it has proven to be of value to the nurse who is striving to
improve her ability to observe through listening. Questions which the
nurse should ask herself are: Was the patient permitted to speak freely
or was his conversation limited by the kinds of questions asked? Were
the questions asked stated in such a way that the patient was encouraged to express himself? Were the patient's responses influenced
by the wording of the question or did he express himself in his own
words? Were both patient and nurse so anxious that they could not
really hear what was being said? Did the patient seem to be trying
to respond in such a way that it seemed he was trying to please the
nurse? What actions or expressions were observed in conjunction with
the comments made? Actually, there may be many more questions to

---

[3]Loretta Sue Bermosk and Mary Jane Mordan, *Interviewing in Nursing* (New
York: The Macmillan Company, 1964), pages 174-178.

be raised by the nurse as she applies this process to her experience. No two interactions are exactly the same, and each will be of value in its own right.

Use of the tape recorder has proven to be of considerable value in the evaluation of a nurse-patient interaction. The recall and recording of a complete account of an interaction is a difficult task, especially when one is unable to write or take notes in the presence of the patient. A tape recording provides a verbatim account of the interview as well as of the periods of silence which can be significant also. As the nurse listens to the tape, she can determine the effectiveness of her approach. For example, a student who recorded an interview with a preoperative patient discovered upon listening to the replay of the tape that she had passed along her own anxious feelings to the patient by suggestion. It was with disbelief that she heard herself ask the patient, "Mrs. X., are you anxious about the surgery you will have?" This experience provided a lasting impression regarding the importance of appropriate questions.

Reviewing a process recording with an instructor provides an opportunity for the instructor to offer helpful suggestions which would not be possible otherwise. The presence of an instructor in the interview situation adds a dimension which may serve as a barrier to communication in that the introduction of a third person may cause the patient to feel uncomfortable about expressing his true thoughts.

INTERPRETATION OF NURSING OBSERVATIONS

Many of the observations to be made by the nurse will be signs and symptoms related to the physical or mental problem of the patient. It is important that significant observations be reported, either verbally or in writing, and that the report be objective. That is, the report should be an account of only what is observed. Such reports of observations serve to assist the physician who will interpret all findings related to the medical problem and subsequently will establish the medical diagnosis. However, the nurse will find that she must be able to interpret her observations to the extent that she must decide what observations are pertinent to the patient's health problem and are therefore significant.

More extensive interpretations of observations will be required in the administration of nursing care to the sick. The nurse must be able to determine first exactly how much assistance is required by the patient. As she continues to minister to the patient, she will need to evaluate the effectiveness of the nursing care given. Continual evaluation of nursing care is essential in order that the changing needs of the patient may be met. For example, when the nurse measures the body temperature of a patient and finds it to be 102 degrees, her action cannot stop with the reporting of her observation. She must recognize the significance of this deviation and must proceed to perform prescribed measures which are directed toward the reduction or control of the temperature. Should she find an order for a specific medication, she would give the medication. In order to determine whether the medication has been effective, the nurse must measure the temperature again when sufficient time has been allowed for the medication to produce its effect. In this case, the nurse interprets her observation of the patient's temperature first as a situation requiring further attention and later as a means of determining whether the nursing care administered has produced the desired effect. This evaluation will enable her to determine what her next move should be.

In any evaluation of the effectiveness of specific nursing care measures, the nurse will be concerned with all observations made including those regarding the specific care rendered and any others related to the total condition of the patient. For example, when a nurse assists a bedfast patient with his preparation for sleep, her objective is to promote comfort and relaxation. In order to achieve this objective, attention will be given to the physical needs of hygiene, elimination, and back care. Also, the bed will be made more comfortable by removing irritants such as crumbs and wrinkles, and by adding sufficient covers to insure warmth. The environment will be prepared by providing for adequate ventilation and by elimination of noise and unnecessary light. In addition, a sedative may be administered in accordance with the orders of the physician. In order to evaluate the effectiveness of all of the aspects of this nursing care, the nurse must observe the patient periodically to determine whether the patient is able to sleep. If she discovers that the patient is unable to sleep, further investigation is necessary to identify the cause of the insomnia. In talking with the patient, the nurse may discover that he is suffering some physical discomfort which requires attention or that he is unable to sleep because of worry or concern about his health problem. The determination of the exact nature of the problem requires the use of knowledge of both the natural and social sciences, in that the nurse must exercise her knowledge of human behavior as well as those facts related to sleep. In a case such as this, the nurse observes for the results of the nursing care directed specifically toward promotion of comfort and sleep. The discovery of a problem which was not solved through the nursing care administered necessitates the consideration or interpretation of all observations surrounding the total situation. While the actual cause of the insomnia may not be one of the areas to which attention has been given, it is still related to the patient's overall condition.

LEARNING THROUGH OBSERVATION

Observation as an aid to learning has been utilized extensively in nursing education. Observation of nursing practice in real or simulated situations provides opportunity for the learner to comprehend more clearly the application of scientific principles in the care of the sick. Observation of nursing practice is made possible through the use of such media as television, films, a practice laboratory, and the actual hospital unit. Study of related scientific principles prior to the experience in observation enhances its value as an aid to learning in that the learner will have more knowledge of specific observations to be made as she sees someone else administer nursing care. A follow up discussion and/or practice session can be of further benefit to the learner in that it provides an opportunity to develop some dexterity before administering the same care to a patient.

As the student progresses, she will discover that observation of the various activities and patients on a hospital unit provides many opportunities for learning. Some patients will exemplify the pathology described in textbooks; problem situations will arise and will demand the expertise of an experienced nurse; and patients will be undergoing many types of therapy all of which are worthy of observation so that the nurse has a better understanding of what the patient is actually experiencing. Whatever the nature of the situation being observed, the student should develop the practice of reflection upon the experience so that she can identify what she has learned through this experience. In so doing, the student should be able to apply this knowledge in future experiences.

OBSERVATION AS A RESEARCH METHOD

With the realization that a clearly defined body of supporting knowledge is a requisite to the practice of a profession, nursing leaders have recognized the pressing need for definition of the specific body of knowledge which supports the practice of nursing and that the only means to accomplish this goal is through concentrated basic and continuous research.[4] Because of the pressing need for this research, nursing curricula are being revised to incorporate an introduction to the theory

---

[4]Martha E. Rogers, *Reveille In Nursing* (New York: The Macmillan Company, 1964), page 11.

and practice of research even in basic professional programs. Graduate programs in nursing education are directed toward the development of skill in the conduct of research. Consequently, it can be anticipated that, as more scientific knowledge is identified, there will be many changes in the practice of nursing, all of which should contribute to improvement in the actual nursing care of the patient. An understanding of the scientific principles involved in the performance of a nursing technique will enable the nurse to adapt that technique to the needs of the individual patient.

While there are several methods which can be utilized in the process of scientific research, the very nature of the nurse-patient relationship provides a unique opportunity for the employment of observation as the method through which data can be collected. As the nurse ministers to the patient consecutively throughout his hospital stay, a recording of her day-to-day observations can provide an invaluable picture of the changes that occur in his total condition. Analysis of such data provides specific information to be used in the evaluation of nursing care measures.

The fact that the nurse participates directly in the care of the patient affords her the opportunity to make many observations which would not be obvious were her role that of a nonparticipant. Awareness that one is being observed can cause a person to behave in a way that might not reveal his true reactions to a situation. Introduction of a third person to serve in the role of observer of a nurse-patient interaction introduces another inhibiting variable which can distort the findings. Because of the importance of validity as a characteristic of research findings, all possible efforts must be taken to reduce such variables. As the nurse works directly with the patient, she can use her skill in the many methods of observation to collect data which can help to prove or disprove the hypothesis set forth in her research design. Although not every nurse will be an expert in research nor will every research project be a major one, it is essential for professional nurses to recognize the value of research findings and their implications for improving nursing care.

IMPORTANCE OF OBSERVATION IN TEAM NURSING

In an attempt to provide a higher quality of nursing care directed toward the total needs of the individual patients, the practice of team nursing has been introduced in many hospital settings. In situations where the implementation of team nursing has been successful, it has proved beneficial to nursing personnel as well as to patients. One of the chief components in the functioning of the successful nursing team is the free communication among all of its members. A part of this communication is the orientation of the team members by their leader who will advise them of significant observations to be made as they administer care to the patient. Another part of this communication occurs in the team conference at which time all members of the team will discuss their observations. Through this sharing of experiences, problems in nursing care can be identified and possible solutions suggested by someone who has encountered similar difficulties in other situations.

The team conference provides an opportunity for all members of the team to learn about the needs of all of the patients for whom the team is responsible. This knowledge enables them to assist one another when necessary. Because of their awareness of special needs of each patient, the patient is spared the frustrating experience of receiving care from someone who is not aware of his limitations or needs. Such experiences cause the patient to feel insecure about the ability of those who are responsible for his care.

Because each day is divided into three eight-hour tours of duty, a written account of observations and problems encountered is essential for the sake of continuity. Each patient has a chart, but its account of all information about the patient makes it too cumbersome to use for quick reference. Consequently, the nursing care plan has come into common usage. This plan provides sufficient information about the specific problems of a patient to enable any member of the nursing team to determine the kind of assistance required by the patient. In order for the nursing care plan to be effective, it must be kept current, that is, as the condition and problems of a patient change, the notations on the care plan must be changed also. It is usually the responsibility of the professional nurse, team leader, or student to keep these plans up-to-date. Nonprofessional personnel communicate their observations to the team leader who then decides what should be recorded on the nursing care plan.

As professional and nonprofessional nursing personnel work together toward the common good of the patient, benefits are afforded patients and nursing personnel. Because the group of nursing personnel is working toward a common goal, they will be inspired by each other with the result that the patient receives better care and the nursing personnel are happier in their work.

SUMMARY

The purpose of the discussion in this chapter has been to demonstrate the importance of observation as a nursing skill which must be employed at all levels of nursing practice. The nurse must possess a knowledge of the natural and social sciences underlying the practice of professional nursing so that she may work with a constant alertness to significant observations.

BIBLIOGRAPHY

BERMOSK, LORETTA SUE, and MORDAN, MARY JANE, *Interviewing in Nursing.* New York: The Macmillan Company, 1964.

FUERST, ELINOR V., and WOLFF, LUVERNE, *Fundamentals of Nursing.* Philadelphia: J. B. Lippincott Company, 1964.

GEORGE, JOYCE HOLMES, "Electronic Monitoring of Vital Signs," *American Journal of Nursing,* Vol. 65, No. 2, 1965, p. 68-71.

HASSENPLUG, LULU WOLF, "Preparation of the Nurse Practitioner," *Journal of Nursing Education,* Vol. 4, No. 1, 1965, p. 29.

KRON, THORA, *Nursing Team Leadership.* Philadelphia: W. B. Saunders Company, 1961.

MACBRYDE, CYRIL MITCHELL, *Signs and Symptoms.* Philadelphia: J. B. Lippincott Company, 1964.

MATHENEY, RUTH V., and others, *Fundamentals of Patient-Centered Nursing.* Philadelphia: J. B. Lippincott Company, 1964.

MCCAIN, R. FAYE, "Nursing by Assessment—Not Intuition," *American Journal of Nursing,* Vol. 65, No. 4, 1965, p. 82.

ROGERS, MARTHA E., *Reveille in Nursing.* New York: The Macmillan Company, 1964.

RUSSELL, C. H., *Liberal Education and Nursing.* New York: Bureau of Publications, Teachers College, Columbia University, 1959.

SKIPPER, JAMES K., and LEONARD, ROBERT C., *Social Interaction and Patient Care.* Philadelphia: J. B. Lippincott Company, 1965.

TOSIELLO, FRANK, "A Liberal Education for Nursing," *Nursing Outlook,* Vol. 13, No. 3, 1965, p. 64-66.

Chapter _____ 2

Observation of Patients
in Their Environment

What does one see when he meets a person for the first time? No doubt the observations made will depend upon the circumstances surrounding the introduction. When meeting someone socially, a person will notice the general appearance with more concern for attractiveness than for the state of health. Such factors as age, neatness, and general body build will be of interest. If concerned with any psychological factors at all, they probably would be more related to the social graces of the individual than to his anxieties. One probably would dismiss without much concern any ideas pertaining to health because this is not the objective of the situation.

In the nursing situation, however, there are different purposes or objectives. The skill of observation is a directed or purposeful consideration of what is being perceived. The nurse must always work with a purpose. When observing a sick person, one looks for characteristics that are different from those which seem predominant in social situations. The observation which the nurse makes as she works with the sick person will be related more directly to his illness and, thus, will be comprised chiefly of the changes resulting from his impaired health conditions. The discussion that follows pertains to some of these specific observations.

POSTURE

The posture assumed by a person is a good indicator of the way he feels, both physically and mentally. To illustrate, if a person is experiencing pain of a particular part of the body, he will carry himself in a manner that protects the affected part. Variations in posture may result also from physical defects such as unequal length of the legs or vertebral defects which interfere with the supportive function of the spine. While some postural defects may be the result of poor habits, patients should be given the benefit of the doubt by calling the observation to the attention of the physician who will determine the cause.

Maintenance of good body posture at all times facilitates such body functions as respiration and circulation. Therefore, it is important that the nurse pay particular attention to the body alignment of patients who cannot help themselves. She should position them so that they have freedom of the air passages, and she should observe them frequently so that they can be assisted into good position relieving the tendency to slump. When helpless patients are assisted into chairs, enough pillows or other supports should be used to enable them to maintain good posture.

ATTITUDES IN ILLNESS

For the purposes of this discussion, the term attitude is used to mean the frame of mind or mental outlook of an individual. The nurse often is asked to describe the patient's state of mind. While this could refer to clarity or orientation, it is used here to mean the mental outlook.

Attitude is one of the first observations made upon being introduced to a new person. It may be whether he is cheerful, depressed, optimistic, pessimistic, or just how he feels about himself and others. By listening to a person talk for a short while and seeking his response to a few key questions, the nurse can learn quite a bit about her patients. Experts in human behavior have demonstrated the effect of illness upon attitude and behavior. They have shown that, during illness, there is a threat to the total person and his self image.[1] For this reason, patients can be expected to express attitudes which may be quite different from their attitudes during periods of good health.

Some ways in which illness poses a threat to the well-being of the individual are to his independence, to his ability to perform his usual activities both vocational and recreational, and to his security, both financial and physical. Changes in attitude may be detected first in the reaction to minor irritations which ordinarily would be brushed off as insignificant. The astute nurse will recognize this signal and will avoid

---

[1]Stanley H. King, *Perceptions of Illness and Medical Practice* (New York: Russell Sage Foundation, 1962), page 211; Sydney Smith, "The Psychology of Illness," *Nursing Forum*, 1964, Vol. III, No. 1, page 35; Ira Davis Trail and J. Victor Monke, "Psyche Sequelae of Surgical Change in Body Structure," *Nursing Forum*, 1963, Vol. II, No. 3, page 20.

the development of barriers to communication such as resentment, anger, and frustration. If at all possible, sources of irritation should be removed from the environment of the patient. For example, if a radio playing nearby seems to annoy the patient, the nurse could suggest that the owner of the radio reduce its volume or close the door to eliminate as much noise as possible. A quiet environment is much more conducive to rest than is one filled with all of the sounds of the hustle and bustle of those in attendance.

Another source of irritation to patients may be visitors. While most people enjoy visiting with others when they feel well, it is very tiresome to the patient in pain or the one who is weak from any type of illness to have a steady stream of visitors. A helpful suggestion would be that the visitors themselves limit the number who come and the length of the visit. Without meaning to be thoughtless or inconsiderate, visitors can make unreasonable demands upon a patient just by their very presence. As a rule, when someone visits in the home, the host or hostess tries to make a pleasant response and, to a certain extent, entertain those who are visiting. The patient may see himself as the host in his hospital room and consequently will exert all of the energy he can muster to entertain those who have come to visit. Many hospitals have adopted lenient rules for visiting hours with the result that visitors tend to spend less time per visit, knowing that they are free to return.

If the nurse observes that the patient appears to be upset by a particular visitor, she should attempt to verify her observation through conversation with the patient. Although it is difficult to deny a close relative the privilege of visiting the patient, a talk with that person either by the nurse or by the physician would provide an opportunity to gain more understanding of the problem. If the nurse or physician can help the relative to understand the patient's problem, efforts to control the length and frequency of visits would be more successful.

Attitudes can be misinterpreted if there is not free communication. If a patient appears to be angry or refuses to cooperate with the hospital, the reason for his behavior should be determined. The patient should be permitted to express himself so that, whenever possible, the irritating factor can be removed. All too often when a patient loses his temper, he is labelled immediately as cross or uncooperative. Fortunately, with the increased understanding of human behavior, nurses are beginning to realize that this is only a mechanism and that the patient is not directing his hostility toward anyone personally. Once the problem is identified and communication is restored, both nurse and patient can focus their attention and energy toward the objective of helping the patient regain his state of health.

Acceptance of the patient as a person with a health problem is vital to effective nursing care. Realizing the effects of illness upon behavior, the nurse often finds it necessary to permit patients to depend upon her for support. It is essential that the nurse keep this in mind and that she avoid looking to the patient for fulfillment of her needs for acceptance and recognition. All too often, patients are classified as being demanding or ungrateful by nurses who do not understand the problems of these patients or the reasons for their behavior.

The attitude of sadness or grief may present problems which are very challenging to the nurse. When a patient does not recover from his illness as smoothly as he had expected or when some further misfortune befalls him, he may become so depressed that he refuses to participate in any activity which has been recommended for him. Grief is especially difficult to handle in the care of the patient with a terminal illness. The difficulty comes because the nurse cannot know exactly how the patient feels and because death is such a final and personal experience that many people face with fear and trepidation. The nurse may be just as fearful of death as is the patient, and it may seem that to ignore the situation is the only solution. However, some patients will want to discuss this problem, perhaps with a clergyman if not with the nurse. Difficult as it is, it is imperative that the nurse give thought and study to the ideas of life and death so that she becomes secure in her own convictions and can offer support to the suffering when the need arises.

The act of crying observed in patients does not necessarily reflect immaturity as is sometimes believed. Crying is a means of relieving tension, and sometimes it is a very beneficial mechanism. Many adults are embarrassed to cry in the presence of others, but the nurse can offer understanding and thus can support the patient through this release of tension. As soon as the patient has regained control, he may be able to face the problem before him with more objectivity. The nurse can help by pointing out the positive factors that should not be overlooked. This becomes more difficult in the care of the patient with a poor prognosis, but guiding the attention of the patient toward those positive aspects of the present day can be helpful in relieving the anxiety. Knowing that someone cares enough to spend some time with him, to help him, to see something worthwhile, can mean a great deal to an anxious patient.

An attitude of indifference is one of the most difficult with which to cope. Such an attitude may be only a front for deeper feelings of concern. By appearing indifferent, the patient can avoid the discomfort of facing problems by denying their existence. Fortunately, this is only temporary, and it is important for the nurse to demonstrate her acceptance of this patient through the care she gives so that when the time arrives that he can express his need for help, he will know where to turn.

While the attitude of joy should not be considered a problem, it, too, can be used as a mechanism for denying one's own problems. There will be times when true happiness is experienced by the hospitalized patient, and he should be permitted to make the most of these experiences. When a patient does not respond to good news with pleasure or happiness, the alert nurse will take the time to determine the reason for the inappropriate response. For example, if a patient seems unhappy at the prospect of going home, it may be because he fears that he will be unable to assume responsibility for his care at home or because he does need help at home but has neither anyone to assume the responsibility nor the means to pay for it. Once the problem is identified, it is quite likely that help can be secured through referral to a public health nursing agency or through the recruitment of a friend or relative who is willing to learn how to give the care that is needed. It is important for the nurse to familiarize herself with the social agencies of the community in which she is working. The church of which the patient is a member should be considered as a possible source of assistance, also. In her efforts to avoid imposition of her religious ideas or beliefs upon a patient, it is very easy for the nurse to overlook this important resource. Many churches have some organized plan of aiding people who are in need. Such information can be obtained through conference with the patient's clergyman. The problem may be one of loneliness for the elderly person who may face his return to an empty home. If this is the case, communication of the problem to interested friends will encourage them to offer assistance.

OBSERVING THE NUTRITIONAL STATUS OF A PATIENT

No nurse is expected to be a nutritionist, but some understanding of nutrition and its importance to good health is essential.[2] When a patient enters the hospital, the nurse should be able to determine by his appearance what his general nutritional status is. The fact that a patient appears heavy and robust does not necessarily mean that he is in good health. The problem of obesity is more serious than the problem of being underweight. As the nurse gains some knowledge of nutrition and

---

[2]Ruth V. Matheney and others, *Fundamentals of Patient-Centered Nursing* (St Louis: The C. V. Mosby Company, 1964), page 165.

of recommended body weights, she will develop some skill in appraising this status.

Color of the skin is a fairly good indicator of the general nutritional state. The skin of the poorly nourished patient is characterized by its pallor, lack of turgor, and pasty appearance. The hair of the malnourished person appears dull and brittle instead of lustrous. As the nurse questions the patient about dietary habits, likes and dislikes, she can determine where to begin working with the problem.

OBSERVING THE VOICE AND SPEECH

Once the mature voice of an individual has developed, marked changes are quite noticeable and usually are an indication of some physical problem. Hoarseness with a subsequent loss of the ability to speak is a rather common companion to upper respiratory infections. When this happens, the nurse can provide her patient with a pad and pencil along with some sort of signalling device and can encourage him to refrain from speaking until his infection has cleared.

Other problems which can produce alteration of the voice may be of a more serious nature which will require prompt attention. Any persistent hoarseness or loss of voice in the absence of concurrent respiratory infection should be brought to the attention of the physician because of its importance as a diagnostic aid in the presence of malignancy involving the larynx.[3] Hoarseness does not necessarily mean that the patient has a malignancy involving his larynx, but in the event that he does, early treatment may mean the difference of several years of life for that person. Although a radical procedure such as a laryngectomy seems to be a catastrophic loss, devices are available which enable people to communicate quite well. Once a patient learns how to use one of these devices, he can get along without too much difficulty.

Esophageal speech is a means of speaking without a special device. This type of speech is produced by swallowing air and then controlling its escape from the stomach so that words can be formed with the mouth as the air is released from the esophagus. Speech by this method is distorted but is recognizable, and the nurse who hears these sounds coming from her patient must avoid expressing shock or amusement at them. The ability to communicate is very important to everyone, and the person who has lost his larynx really appreciates the value of communication. The nurse should ascertain what progress the patient is making and can offer further assistance by referring him to the nearest Lost Chord Club where he can meet others who have the same handicap.

---

[3]American Cancer Society, A *Cancer Source Book for Nurses*, 1963, page 69.

This organization has chapters located in many cities across the country; their chief aim is to help those who must learn to live without a larynx to make this adjustment.

General tone of the voice is another quality worthy of observation. Normally, the feminine voice is soft and high-pitched whereas the masculine voice is deep and of strong character. In some metabolic and endocrine disturbances, marked changes occur with the result that a woman might develop a very deep, masculine voice and vice versa. When this happens, the patient is likely to be embarrassed by what has happened to him. He will need as much support as the nurse can give him to keep him from withdrawing into the seclusion of his room. An attitude of acceptance of the individual can do more to offer moral support than many words which are spoken casually.

Further consideration should be given to the matter of speech, that is, the quality of speech. The use of correct grammar is of much less importance than the quality of speech which results from some type of impediment. Some of the impediments which can be detected most easily are, slurring of words, difficulty in word formation, stuttering, and inability to complete sentences.

Of the impediments mentioned, some have a physiologic cause while others may be the result of other problems. Slurring of speech occurs frequently in patients who have experienced brain insult, either permanent or temporary. In any event, patients who have difficulty speaking and making their needs known become very frustrated individuals. Nurses working with them must exercise unlimited patience to help them find some way to express themselves. Much work has been done in recent years to develop aids for people who are handicapped by aphasia. Methods have been devised whereby some of these people can be taught to speak again.[4] Since this learning must begin at the very simple formation of words and sounds, a great deal of time and perseverance is required. In order to do this, there are now skilled speech therapists who spend their entire days helping patients learn to speak again. Some of them work with children who have never been able to speak before, and many of them work with adults who are in need of rehabilitation.

Whenever a nurse works with a patient who is receiving speech therapy, it would be beneficial to her and to the patient if she would accompany the patient for his therapy periodically so that she could observe the work of the patient and the therapist. She would be able, then, to reinforce the therapy through her opportunities to talk with

---

[4]Elizabeth W. Reeves, "The Aphasic Patient," *Nursing Outlook,* Vol. 11, No. 7, 1963, page 522.

the patient, thus stimulating him to practice his work. Because these patients become discouraged easily, they need a great deal of encouragement from the nurse. The family should be invited to participate in this process also, so that they, too, can learn to communicate with the patient.

Patients with more transient or limited problems with speech require precise observation also. The detailed account of events can be very significant in the determination of the cause of the problem. This is especially important in the care of the elderly patient who may be subject to circulatory problems which interfere with the blood supply to the area of the brain controlling speech. Changes in speech may be the only noticeable symptom as mild attacks occur.

As one works with people, it becomes possible to make some assessment of the general type of personality of people by their manner of speech. It has been demonstrated by the experts in dynamics of behavior that very loud, boisterous people who constantly call attention to themselves are doing this in an effort to overcome their insecurity. People who have self-confidence usually are able to speak in a well-controlled and modulated manner. While these observations may not always apply, they at least represent some pertinent observations that can be made.

OBSERVING THE EYES

Quite naturally, the first thought about observation of the eyes is of their primary function, that of sight. Because vision is vitally important, all necessary attention should be given to insure protection and maintenance of this function. Only the patient is able to define exactly what he can or cannot see, but there may be warnings of problems about which he does not know. A person can be squinting as he reads without realizing that he is doing so. Also, signs and symptoms of serious problems involving the eyes may be present but may go unrecognized by those who know nothing of the many diseases that can affect the eye.

The eyes may serve as warning signals to disorders of other parts of the body, also. Some of the changes that take place may be seen only by the physician as he examines the eye with the ophthalmoscope. But there are some changes that are detectable with the naked eye. One of the most common is change in the color of the sclera. Normally, the sclera is the whitest part of the body and, for this reason, it is often the first place that the yellow discoloration which signals the problem of jaundice can be seen. Jaundice is only a sign, but when it is seen, it provides evidence that the pigments which are released in the breakdown of red blood cells are not being excreted through the bile as they should be.[5] This change in color can be seen best in the daylight, but as the condition progresses, it can be seen even in artificial light. When the nurse is caring for patients with any type of liver disease or blood dyscrasia, she should be alert to the development of this problem.

Redness of the sclera has many meanings ranging from sleepiness to serious infections. Any persistent redness of the sclera should be checked by the physician so that therapy can be instituted. Eye infections are especially difficult to handle because of the poor blood supply to the sclera itself. Before making her report, the nurse should ascertain whether the redness is accompanied by itching, pain, or discharge. The presence of a discharge or drainage from the eye should signal the nurse to the existence of some problem. The drainage may be excessive tearing, or it may have the characteristics of drainage from any site of infection.

The importance of protecting the eyes from contamination cannot be overemphasized. Because of their proximity to each other, there is a great potential for cross contamination. It is for this reason that drops are inserted from the inner canthus as the patient turns his head away from the dropper. Irrigations, when ordered, are performed in the same manner. The patient should be taught to keep his hands away from his eyes so that he does not introduce additional infection.

When caring for patients with neurological disorders, there are some symptoms that can be seen in the eye. This is particularly true of any patient who has suffered a head injury which may be causing an increase in intracranial pressure. Eye changes that may be seen are changes in the size of the pupils and variations in their ability to react to light. The nurse will be asked to check the eyes periodically to evaluate their status. A flashlight may be required to detect the condition of inequality in the size of the pupils or inability to react to light.

Generally, the eyes play an important role in facial expression. Although facial expression is not directly related to pathology, the mood of the patient is sometimes quite relevant to his illness. The eyes reflect attitudes of happiness, anxiety, worry, apprehension, and depression. Therefore, the nurse should learn to recognize these characteristics, too.

OBSERVING GAIT

Walking is one of the earliest skills that man develops and, one might say, one of the most essential. Because of the unsteadiness of their gait in beginning experiences, children may have problems in-

---

[5]Jean C. Barbata, Deborah M. Jensen and William G. Patterson, *A Textbook of Medical-Surgical Nursing* (New York: G. P. Putnam's Sons, 1964), page 464.

volving the musculoskeletal system which go unnoticed for quite a while. Most gross abnormalities are detected early, but it is important to observe closely the child who is beginning to walk so that mild problems can be corrected.

In the adult, there are many medical problems which can affect the way in which a person walks. They may be degenerative or infectious disorders. Some may involve primarily the musculoskeletal system, while others may involve the nervous system. Some may occur as a result of weakness which is caused by some other type of illness. Such adjectives as shuffling, staggering, and limping may be used to describe the way a person walks. The nurse should take note of the way ambulatory patients walk. She should notice whether they are able to walk with a fairly erect posture and in a balanced pattern or if they are in need of any kind of support to maintain equilibrium as they navigate from one area to another.

Sometimes it is possible to determine the presence of pain by the way in which a person walks. The patient who is experiencing pain in any part of his body will make an effort to protect that part from strain as he walks. This is a response that occurs without deliberate thought. If a patient is observed walking in a stooped manner, he should be questioned to determine whether he is experiencing back pain. Because of its role in supporting the body weight, the back is a frequent source of discomfort. Prompt attention should be given to this problem so that further injury can be prevented.

Shuffling or loss of control of the feet can be seen in patients who are suffering circulatory problems which have interfered with the proper functioning of the nervous system or from problems which involve the nervous system directly. Also, patients who are bedfast for long periods without exercise of their feet and legs can lose muscle tone with a resulting footdrop which becomes difficult to correct once activity is resumed. For this reason, nurses should protect the feet of bedfast patients from the weight of heavy covers. Range of motion exercises should be utilized to help maintain tone of muscles that must lie quietly for extended periods. Judgment must be exercised in the administration of this aspect of nursing care, however. Patients who have suffered fractures of their feet or legs may be required to have these parts immobilized to insure skeletal healing. If the nurse is in doubt, she can always consult the physician before exercising her patients. It must be remembered, also, that range of motion exercises do not consist of vigorous and strenuous exercise but involve only the action which simulates the normal movement of the part without undue strain.

Limping is a symptom which can be observed in people at any age. It can be seen in people who have pain in a specific part or in patients who have problems in the formation of the skeletal system. Limping occurs as a protective mechanism and, if the problem which is causing it is not corrected, more serious problems involving the entire supportive structure of the body can develop. Limping can be so mild that it goes unnoticed by those who are in closest contact with a person. It should be mentioned that limps can be affected as mechanisms to attract attention. However, the wise nurse will hesitate to draw this conclusion until the patient has been given the benefit of medical examination.

When patients are learning to walk following fractures of any of the bones in the leg, they may be taught special gaits to use with canes or crutches.[6] Variations in gait may be required when a person must learn to walk with a cast, also. Once the injury has healed and the aids are removed, it is important that the nurse help the patient concentrate upon regaining a posture which does not produce undue strain on any part of the body.

OBSERVING APPETITE AND FLUID INTAKE

Food and water are just as essential for the maintenance of body function for the sick person as for the well person.[7] The type of diet the patient should receive is one of the first questions that the nurse will have when a new patient is admitted. Once the order for diet has been obtained and provision is made for the patient's water supply, the nurse's responsibility for observing begins. It is not enough to set a tray in front of a patient and leave him to his own devices. The nurse must determine whether this patient requires assistance with his food. Assistance required may range from convenient placement and cutting of meat to actual feeding. As the nurse helps the patient with his food, she can learn from the patient about any particular food likes or dislikes. Any problems with allergies should be noted, also. The nurse can assess the patient's ability to cope with the food which he is served. If he has poor dentition, it may be necessary to order a type of diet which requires less chewing.

It is important to observe the amount of food consumed by the patient. In the case of measured portions, as for the diabetic patient, it is particularly important to observe whether the patient has con-

---

[6]*Ibid.*, pages 664-665.

[7]Matheney and others, *op. cit.*, pages 165-180; 250-268; 286-292.

sumed his entire meal. If he has not, there may be danger of his reacting later to the insulin which he has received. Because of this, these patients are encouraged to try to eat the recommended portions. If they are unable to do so, replacement may have to be provided through some other means.

Amount of fluid consumed should be observed, also. In some cases, it will be necessary to measure the fluid consumed and to keep an accurate record of this intake. Sometimes, it will be desirable to limit fluids, while, at other times, it may be necessary to persuade patients to drink more. The differences in recommended fluid intake are influenced by the type of medical problem for which the patient is being treated. Whenever fluids are to be restricted for any reason, the information should be communicated to the patient and to all who are concerned with his care. To insure proper management of the patient, the nurse must become familiar with the system used to signify special restrictions, whether it is by a card attached to the bed, by a color-coded marker, or simply through the use of the kardex.

OBSERVING ELIMINATION

Elimination is a basic need of all people, and maintenance of a healthy state is dependent upon it.[8] If the waste products from the normal metabolic processes are not excreted, the patient can develop serious problems. It is known that some fluids and waste products are excreted through the skin and respirations. While the exact amounts cannot be measured, except in extremely well-controlled situations, the fact that this excretion occurs and is essential cannot be disputed.

It is the purpose here, however, to consider those aspects of elimination which can be measured or evaluated, that is, elimination by means of the bowel and bladder. Inhabitants of this country are chided frequently for their extreme interest in bowel function and for the appalling amounts of laxatives consumed. It is known that each individual must establish his own pattern for elimination, and the important consideration is that it be maintained. Much emphasis was formerly placed upon the use of laxatives and enemas for patients, particularly those who were being treated surgically. Some surgeons have initiated the practice of using these artificial devices only when a portion of the digestive tract will be affected directly by the surgery. That is, patients having other than abdominal surgery may be permitted to reestablish their own pattern of elimination when they become active

_____

[8]*Ibid.*, pages 165-180.

and are able to eat again. The exercise of early ambulation makes this type of management more feasible than the bedrest which formerly was required for such long periods.

Nurses have been the subject of many criticisms because of their daily ritual of inquiring as to the bowel function of their patients. Since elimination is essential, it is important for the nurse to ascertain whether her patients are experiencing any problems with this function. It is known that such factors as change in environment, food, and activity will influence elimination. If, through her inquiry, the nurse learns that a patient is having a problem, this problem can be called to the attention of the physician who will in turn prescribe appropriate therapy.

If a patient is having diarrhea, the nurse should ask the patient to collect a specimen in a container provided so that examination for presence of mucus or blood could be noted. Also, when a patient has diarrhea it is important to record the number and frequency of bowel movements. If this condition is allowed to persist, the patient may lose important electrolytes which will necessitate replacement.

Color and consistency of the feces becomes particularly important in the care of patients with such problems as gall bladder disease and problems of bleeding as from peptic ulcers. In the presence of obstruction of the biliary tract of a patient, the feces assume a clay color because of the inability of the body to excrete bile into the intestinal tract. Bile normally gives the stool its brownish color. When there is bleeding in the stomach or duodenum, the stool may take on a tarry color and a jelly-like consistency. This is caused by the digestion of the blood as it is exposed to the digestive juices. In the presence of disturbance in the patient's ability to digest fats, the stool may take on a fatty appearance and may emit a most noxious odor.

The most frequent observations of the urinary output are related to the amount. The amount excreted daily varies among individuals, but it is known to be influenced both by fluid intake and kidney function. Some of the patients who most commonly require measurement of fluid output include those with some types of circulatory problems, those who have just had surgery, those with problems of the genitourinary tract, those with certain kinds of endocrine dysfunction, and patients who have experienced extensive trauma. Whenever it is necessary to keep a record of urinary output, every effort should be made to keep the record accurately. Unless the patient is disoriented or unconscious, he should be instructed as to the importance of this activity, and his cooperation must be requested. Some terms commonly used to describe variations in the amount of urinary output are: anuria, which means the absence of urinary output; oliguria, which means a scant or diminished amount of urinary output; and polyuria, which refers to increased or an excessive amount of urinary output.

In addition to observing the amount of urine excreted by the patient, the nurse should take note of any peculiar characteristic such as cloudiness, color other than the normal straw color, and unusual odor. The presence of blood in the urine is referred to as hematuria. Odor becomes especially significant in the care of patients with diabetes and in those who have urinary tract infections. If a patient with diabetes is spilling acetone into his urine as a result of his metabolic disequilibrium and incomplete fat metabolism, his urine will have an odor which is described, characteristically, as fruit-like.

Some patients may have difficulty in expelling urine. If this is suspected by the scant amount of urine voided, the nurse should check the patient's abdomen to see if his urinary bladder seems distended. The nurse can learn to palpate the area just above the symphysis pubis. If distention is present, the bladder will be palpable as a hard, rounded mass.

If it is necessary for a patient to have a catheter inserted for urinary drainage, the nurse must observe the tubing to be sure that it is not obstructed in any way. Irrigations may be ordered to maintain the patency of this tubing. It should be remembered that the drainage system leading from the urethra to a receptacle should be handled with sterile technique to prevent pathogenic organisms from entering the tubing and ascending into the bladder. Observations of a break in this technique should be followed by replacement of the contaminated equipment.

OBSERVING SLEEP

Observing a person as he sleeps can tell the nurse many things about the condition of that person. If he is only dozing, he may be uncomfortable from an uncomfortable bed, from worries that may be on his mind, or from pain which he has not admitted. Because sleep and rest are essential for good body function, it is important to see to it that the patient gets an adequate amount of rest while he is in the hospital.[9] In illness, the need for sleep may be increased so that body energy can be utilized for the healing process rather than in physical activity.

Characteristics of sleep may vary from a light sleep which is broken frequently to a deep sleep which may last for several consecutive hours. It is important to know whether the patient appears to be able to relax and get to sleep readily or if he needs sedation to induce sleep. People react differently to being in the hospital or just to being away from

---

[9]*Ibid.,* pages 156-164.

home. Some can sleep without difficulty, but others may find that their illness coupled with a strange bed and environment make it difficult for them to sleep.

It is a commonly known fact that the night is the longest and most dreaded part of the day for people who are ill. Although patients may yearn for a little quiet during the hustle and bustle of the busy day, the still, dark, solitude of the night can seem almost unbearable. It is essential, therefore, that the nurse be aware of the sleep habits of her patients and that she recognize their needs for care during the night. Nursing care required may consist only of companionship and a listening ear, or it may be attention to vital machines that must operate continuously. Sometimes, a backrub, change of position, drink of water, or fluffing of the pillow may have a more relaxing effect than a sedative.

When sedatives are given, it is important to realize that people do react differently to these medications. Small doses given to one person may produce a long, uninterrupted sleep, whereas the same amount given to someone else may produce little or no effect. Then, there will be some patients who react in the most unexpected way in that they are stimulated by sedatives rather than relaxed by them. In such cases, confusion is a possibility, and safety precautions should be taken to protect the patient from falling or injuring himself in some other way. Such confusion occurs especially in elderly patients who seem to be less able to tolerate drugs.

When patients have been given sedatives, the nurse should observe the kind of sleep that follows. One way of telling whether the patient is relaxed is by looking at his facial expression. If his face appears to be at ease, he is probably resting well, but if he is wearing a grimace, there is a likelihood that he is having pain and that he is not really sleeping as desired. Because patients react differently to light and sound while sleeping, people working during the night must try to work as quietly as possible to avoid unnecessary disturbances.

Reporting observations of patients' sleep should consist of more than a sketchy "sleeping" or "resting quietly" as may be seen on nurses' notes. It is important to be specific about the characteristics of the sleep so that the physician reading the notes can ascertain whether his patient is responding to therapy or whether he should have some other medication prescribed.

OBSERVING PROSTHESES

Whenever a patient enters the hospital wearing a prosthesis of any sort, the nurse should observe not only its presence but also its effectiveness, that is, the way it fits and whether it is causing any irritation.

From the patient, the nurse can learn what care the prosthesis requires or what care the patient has been giving it. Additional instructions may be required to help the patient learn proper care. Any special equipment necessary for the care of the prosthesis should be provided for the patient. This applies to artificial eyes, dentures, and artificial limbs. Provision should be made for artificial limbs and any canes or crutches used in walking to be kept within easy reach of a patient who is permitted out of bed.

OBSERVING STATE OF ORIENTATION AND LEVELS OF CONSCIOUSNESS

Because so many illnesses produce changes in the ability of patients to respond to stimuli, the nurse should make some assessment of the degree of orientation of her patients.[10] Many patients will be quite alert and clearly oriented, but patients with head injuries, toxic conditions, or those who are experiencing the degenerative changes which occur with old age may show signs of confusion. When patients are unconscious for any reason, the nurse will be expected to observe closely for changes in the level of consciousness. Some patients may respond to no stimuli, not even painful ones. Patients who do not respond even to painful stimuli must be considered to be critically ill, and they will most often be found in the intensive care unit, if the hospital is equipped with one. Constant care is required for such patients so that assistance will be available for the maintenance of the vital functions of respiration and circulation.

Some patients will be unconscious but will show response to such stimuli as movement and light. When patients have had brain surgery or trauma, the nurse will be expected to check the response of the pupils to light. The response or lack of it serves as a guide to the development of increased pressure within the cranium. This pressure might be increasing as a result of edema or bleeding. In either event, its detection is important.

There will be some patients who appear to be sleeping most of the time but who will respond when commands are given. It is important to determine whether their response seems clear or confused. The word sensorium is used to mean the clarity of mind or degree of orientation of a person. It may be described as clear if the person is aware of his whereabouts and cloudy if he seems confused about time or place. Observation of the level of consciousness and orientation should be made

---

[10]*Ibid.*, page 221.

periodically to determine whether the patient seems lucid at intervals and confused at others.

When patients have major surgery, they are rendered unconscious by the use of anesthetics. It is important to observe the level of consciousness as these patients gradually recover from the anesthetic effect of the drug given. The progression back to consciousness demonstrates the various levels of consciousness from the absence of response to external stimuli to the state of awareness and alertness.

The unconscious patient is completely dependent upon the nurse, and only through her surveillance will she detect problems that might jeopardize his well-being. Perhaps the problem of most importance is that of maintaining an open airway. The head of the unconscious patient must be kept in a position that will insure an open airway. If an unconscious patient vomits, the nurse must act quickly to turn his head to the side so that the material will not be aspirated into the lungs where it can cause obstruction and pneumonia.

Care of the skin becomes increasingly important for the unconscious patient. Since he is unable to exercise and change his position voluntarily, it is possible for certain areas of the body to be subjected to continuous pressure which can be traumatic to the tissue. Areas of particular importance are those where bony prominences appear. Because of the proximity of the bone to the skin in these areas, the subcutaneous tissues are subjected to damaging pressure when one position of the patient is maintained for long periods of time. Skin damaged by such pressure may break down, and decubitus ulcers may form. When this occurs in patients who have already suffered severe body insult, the healing process is slow and can become quite complicated. Therefore, the skin of the unconscious patient should be protected through proper cleansing, application of a lubricating body lotion, and frequent changes in position with due caution for protection of bony prominences from pressure. The use of pillows or other soft materials may be indicated to protect areas from pressure and from the prolonged contact of skin and bedding surfaces.

OBSERVING THE ENVIRONMENT

Observation of the immediate environment can be as important as observation of the patient. One objective of nursing care is to promote comfort of the patient; another is to insure safety of the patient. When the nurse works with an awareness of these objectives, she sees beyond the patient and his bed to notice other factors which may influence the achievement of these objectives.

There are several things the nurse can do to make the unit or room of the patient more safe and comfortable. Proper ventilation will improve the atmosphere of the room by introducing fresh air and permitting stale or unpleasant odors to escape. Caution is necessary to protect the patient from drafts, however. Odors which persist even though the room is ventilated can be controlled by other means. There are several types of room deodorants and deodorizers available. Some of the wick type deodorants are quite effective. There are machines available, too, which act as deodorizers. Regardless of the type chosen, some kind of deodorant should be used when an unpleasant odor is present. Removal of the cause of the odor is the most desirable method of control but, in some instances, this is not possible.

The nurse should assist the patient who requires help into a position which is comfortable and which maintains good body alignment. It must be remembered that the position of the patient should be changed periodically, since even the most comfortable positions become tiresome if they are maintained too long. An abundance of pillows will be helpful, too, in promoting the comfort of the bedfast patient. Soft pillows can be just as supportive as hard ones and can offer much more comfort.

Among the basic needs of every individual is the need for safety.[11] This need assumes even greater importance for the person who is unable to help himself. As the person responsible for the safety of the patient, the nurse must be alert to any potential safety hazards in the hospital environment. The removal of safety hazards from a patient's unit or room is important in the prevention of injuries to patients. The prevention of injuries to other hospital personnel is important, also. Such hazards as handles used for raising and lowering beds and casters should be kept in such a position that no one will trip over them or bump into them. Anything that has been dropped or spilled on the floor should be cleaned up immediately so that a patient or nurse does not slip and sustain serious injury. The patient's bedside stand should be left close enough to the bed to permit the patient to reach it for any of his belongings. Otherwise, a patient can fall from his bed as he attempts to get the things he needs without calling someone to help. Electrical equipment and cords must be in good condition and must be protected from damage which might, in turn, result in fire.

Fire is always a hazard in the hospital, and for this reason, smokers should be provided with proper equipment for disposal of ashes and other waste material. When bedfast patients are permitted to smoke, enough assistance should be provided to prevent accidents. The nurse

---

[11]A. H. Maslow, *Motivation and Personality* (New York: Harper and Brothers, 1954), pages 80-92.

should familiarize herself with the overall plan for action if a fire does occur in the hospital. She must know where the equipment which can be used to fight fire is kept, how to send for help, how to recognize the signals of fire occurring in other areas, and the procedure for evacuation when necessary.

When patients are permitted to be up and about, the room should contain only the essential furniture and equipment. Pathways to the door and to the bathroom should be kept clear at all times. Most hospitals have night lights which offer some protection to patients who must get up during the night.

Noise is probably one of the most difficult of all problems in the hospital environment. With the emphasis upon sanitation, hospitals have been constructed of materials which lend themselves to easy maintenance. Unfortunately, these materials tend to act as amplifiers rather than absorbing noise, and the patient who is trying so desperately to rest finds himself being stimulated almost constantly from what almost seems to be uncontrollable noise. There are some ways in which noise can be reduced, however, such as thoughtfulness of personnel in speaking, the careful use of equipment, and control of radio and television equipment in the area. Patients should not be denied the pleasure derived through the media of radio and television. Their days and nights are long, and any enjoyable diversion should be permitted. The use of individual speaker sets which fit nicely under or upon the pillow reduce considerably the noise emitted into the hallways to echo from one room to another. Some hospitals now require that any television sets used in the patient's room be equipped with these devices.

Maintenance of equipment is a must in order to insure the safety of the patient. The nurse must recognize defects in the operation of such equipment as wheelchairs, lounge chairs, or stretchers and must see to it that proper repairs are made promptly. Electrical equipment should be inspected periodically so that defective cords or any other parts can be replaced.

Although the nurse should not be responsible for floor cleaning, she should report any spilled liquid to the appropriate person so that the hazard can be removed. There may be fragments of glass on the floor also, and when the nurse sees these, she should see to it that they are removed. Patients sometimes wear rather soft and thin slippers which could be pierced by sharp fragments of glass.

If a patient has treatments in process such as intravenous therapy or oxygen therapy, the nurse must learn to look for any problem in the administration of these treatments. At a glance, the nurse should discern whether the intravenous fluids are running properly and if a new bottle is needed. By looking at the appropriate gauge, she can determine exactly how much oxygen a patient is receiving. If a patient is receiving oxygen by tent, the nurse must be able to tell at a glance whether the tent is secured properly. Drainage bottles of any sort should be checked as often as the nurse passes a patient's unit.

This kind of checking can be done frequently and without specifically timed visits to the unit if the nurse is aware of the needs of her patients. While the beginner in nursing may not be able to look for all of these things as she enters her patient's room, with concentrated effort, this ability can be developed as her confidence grows in the performance of the various nursing functions.

SUMMARY

Observation of patients in a hospital setting encompasses all of the observations which are related specifically to the patient's physical and general psychological condition. This chapter has been devoted to a discussion of what to observe in order to evaluate the human body and its key physiologic functions. An understanding of human behavior and the factors which affect it is essential to observation of a person during illness. Since a part of the nurse's responsibility is to provide a therapeutic environment, it is essential that she be alert to the development of irritating factors which interfere with the comfort and safety of the patient.

BIBLIOGRAPHY

ABERG, HARRIET, "The Nurse's Role in Hospital Safety," *Nursing Outlook*, Vol. 5, No. 3, 1957, p. 160-162.

BARBATA, JEAN C., JENSEN, DEBORAH M., and PATTERSON, WILLIAM G., *A Textbook of Medical-Surgical Nursing.* New York: G. P. Putnam's Sons, 1964.

CONNALLY, MARY GRACE, "What Acceptance Means to Patients," *American Journal of Nursing*, Vol. 60, No. 12, 1960, p. 1754-1757.

MATHENEY, RUTH V., and others, *Fundamentals of Patient-Centered Nursing.* St. Louis: The C. V. Mosby Company, 1964.

REEVES, ELIZABETH W., "The Aphasic Patient," *Nursing Outlook*, Vol. 11, No. 7, 1963, p. 522.

SMITH, DOROTHY W., and GIPS, CLAUDIA D., *Care of the Adult Patient*, 2nd ed. Philadelphia: J. B. Lippincott Company, 1966.

STEVENS, LEONARD F., "What Makes A Ward Climate Therapeutic?" *American Journal of Nursing*, Vol. 61, No. 3, 1961, p. 95-96.

TRAIL, IRA, and MONKE, J. VICTOR, "Psyche Sequelae of Surgical Change in Body Structure." *Nursing Forum*, Vol. II, No. 3, 1963, p. 20.

WESTBERG, GRANGER, *Nurse, Pastor and Patient.* Rock Island, Illinois: Augustana Press, 1955.

Chapter _____ 3

Observation of Signs
and Symptoms

Although the nurse is taught to recognize symptoms, she must realize that they are symptoms and that her task is not to establish a medical diagnosis but is simply to report what she sees. In reporting her observations, she must be accurate and concise, avoiding expressions of opinion or medical interpretation. There will be instances, however, when the nurse must interpret observations that have direct influence upon the care she must give to the patient. These interpretations are related more specifically to the kind of nursing assistance the patient will require as a result of his illness.

DEFINITION OF SYMPTOMS

To define symptom, the further classification into objective and subjective symptoms is used.[1] For the purposes of this book, the term, objective symptoms, will be used to include any visible or measurable sign of variation from the normal state of health or usual pattern of behavior. This means that the phrase objective symptoms is considered to be synonymous with signs. Objective symptoms or signs are those guides which ordinarily are spoken of as the vital signs, that is, pulse rate, respiratory rate, blood pressure, and, in some instances, body temperature as well as changes in the appearance of any part of the body or the behavior of the patient. Clear and concise descriptions of observations enable the one who is receiving the report to develop an overall image of the state of events. This report may be included as

---

[1]Cyril Mitchell MacBryde, *Signs and Symptoms* (Philadelphia: J. B. Lippincott Company, 1964), page 1.

a part of the nursing notes, or it may be presented verbally to another nurse or to the physician.

Subjective symptoms are those symptoms which the patient feels but which have no external manifestation. Common examples of this type of symptom are pain, numbness, itching, and the like. Because of the extent to which the nurse must rely upon the patient for a description of these symptoms, precautions must be taken to insure accurate reports. It is common knowledge that the power of suggestion can influence behavior and expression. The use of qualifying adjectives should be avoided when attempting to ascertain from the patient how he feels. A more accurate picture will be obtained if the patient is allowed to describe what he feels in his own words. If necessary, the nurse can translate these words into the terminology that is used more commonly by the nursing and medical professions.

OBSERVING THE VITAL SIGNS

Among the most frequently requested observations are those which are generally referred to as the vital signs. The term vital indicates the importance of these signs as guides to the total condition of a patient.

The request for vital signs to be recorded at periodic intervals means that the pulse and respiratory rates and the blood pressure reading should be determined as often as specified. In some cases, the term vital signs may include a reading of the body temperature also. Ordinarily, however, temperature is not ordered to be checked as often as the other signs listed above. A graphic record is kept of the periodic readings, and any additional observations should be recorded in the nurses' notes. There are several factors which should be observed about each one of these signs.

The rate of the pulse is one of the first observations to be made when patients enter the hospital or are stricken by illness. The pulse is counted most frequently at the point where the radial artery lies along the medial aspect of the distal end of the radius. The pulse is palpable at several other areas where an artery is near the surface of the body with a bone in back of the artery to offer support when mild pressure is exerted. These areas are: (1) the point at which the temporal artery passes just in front of the ear or slightly higher almost in line with the crest of the eyebrow; (2) the site where the femoral artery passes through the groin; (3) the point in the back of the knee where the popliteal artery lies near the surface; and (4) the site at which the pedal artery can be palpated over the fourth metatarsal bone, just behind the fourth toe.

There are several variations which may occur in the pulse rate. Normally, the pulse rate will range between sixty and ninety beats per minute with the rate of the female usually being somewhat more rapid than that of the male. The name for a very rapid pulse is tachycardia, while a very slow pulse is bradycardia. Pulse rate is especially significant in patients who suffer heart disease and are being treated with the drug digitalis or one of its derivatives.[2] The action of digitalis is to produce stronger and more regular contractions of the ventricles. An additional effect is a reduction in the pulse rate. Since this reduction in rate may have some bearing upon the amount of drug which the patient should receive, the pulse is counted both radially and over the apex of the heart before administering a dose of the drug. The general rule is that if the pulse is below sixty, the physician should be consulted before administering the drug.

In order to obtain an accurate determination of the apical and radial pulses, two nurses are required to observe and count the two simultaneously. The reason for this type of measurement is to detect the occurrence of ventricular contractions that are too weak to send a pulse wave to the radial artery. When such contractions occur, there will be a difference in the rate of the two pulses. This difference is called pulse deficit. It is determined by subtracting the radial pulse from the apical pulse.

In addition to counting the rate of the pulse, its quality and rhythm should be observed. The pulse relays certain information about the heart, since it is produced by the contraction of the ventricles. For this reason, it is possible to determine whether the heart is contracting rhythmically or if there is interruption in its rhythm. Deviations in rhythm may vary from an occasional missed beat to a pattern of periodic misses. One rather striking type of irregularity is called a gallop rhythm. This means that there is a pattern which has a rhythm similar to the rhythmic clatter heard when a horse gallops. If irregularity is detected, it should be reported with a description of the rhythm palpated.

The quality of the pulse reflects the force with which the blood is being pumped through the arteries. When a patient is in a state of good health, there would be a strong pulse with a regular rhythm. If a patient is in a state of shock, the pulse becomes weak and the rhythm may or may not be discernible. A pulse of such weak quality is referred to as thready pulse, in that all of the pulsations seem to run along as a continuous thread with very small knots in it. In some in-

---

[2]Elsie E. Krug, *Pharmacology in Nursing*, 9th ed. (St. Louis: The C. V. Mosby Company, 1963), page 427.

stances, the pulse may seem to be bounding in quality. Again, deviation should be recorded.

Since the body depends upon the respiratory function of the lungs to provide sufficient oxygen to carry on its processes, it is essential that an adequate respiratory pattern be maintained. If, for some reason, a person is unable to perform this function adequately, assistance may be required. Assistance required may vary from maintaining a position which facilitates breathing to using a mechanical device which literally breathes for the patient. An example of the importance of position can be seen in the patient who has shortness of breath which is relieved by sitting in an upright position. When such a patient is permitted to slump, the difficulty in breathing is increased. The nurse must observe the position of such patients frequently and must take appropriate steps to promote respiratory function.

Variations in the respirations of most patients will be related to the rate and depth. Breathing is considered to be an involuntary function; in the usual state of good health, respiration occurs without any deliberate effort on the part of the patient. This, of course, refers to the breathing of a person who is either at rest or performing ordinary activity which does not produce exertion. When the patient performs strenuous activities, such as running or climbing stairs, which increase the demand for oxygen, the respiratory rate and depth increase to meet this demand. Except in special situations such as specific tests of the patient's breathing capacity, the nurse will be counting the respirations while the patient is at rest. Considerable variation in the respiratory rates of different people will be observed, with the majority occurring in the range from 16 to 20 respirations per minute. The respiratory rate rises with increase in body temperature and pulse rate in order to provide enough oxygen to meet the demands of increased metabolic rate. Certain drugs, such as hypnotics and potent analgesics, produce depression of the vital centers in the central nervous system with a resultant decrease in respiratory rate. For this reason, the nurse is advised to determine the rate of respirations before administering medications which are known to produce this effect.

Some variations which may be noticed in the respiratory patterns of the sick are: (1) dyspnea, any difficulty in breathing which is the body's attempt to increase the amount of oxygen available to the blood as it passes thorugh the lungs and is characterized by labored respirations or shortness of breath; (2) apnea, the temporary cessation of respiration which is restored either by natural or artificial means; (3) hyperpnea, rapid respirations as may be seen after strenuous activity; (4) oligopnea, slow respirations as seen in response to morphine or other central nervous system depressants: (5) orthopnea, difficulty with respirations which requires the patient to assume a sitting position to breathe; and (6) Cheyne Stokes Respirations which are characterized by alternate periods of apnea and shallow respirations. Cheyne Stokes respirations are usually an indication of serious cerebral disturbance and they are most often seen in the terminally ill patient.

Depth of respirations merits observation also. While no one breathes at his full vital capacity during a normal respiratory cycle, the supply of oxygen to the body is dependent upon the depth of respirations. Actually, the entire breathing space is not needed for respiration under normal conditions. The body can obtain adequate oxygen supply when only one lung is functioning, but the failure to use the remaining lung tissue can be harmful to that tissue. When the lungs are not being expanded for deep respirations, there is a danger of obstruction in the bronchial tree which leads to the unused portion. This obstruction occurs as a result of the collection of mucus which is not being carried out into the bronchi for excretion via coughing or swallowing. An example of this situation is the postoperative patient who has been lying quietly in the same position for several hours. Because of the danger of fluid collection and inadequate inflation of the lungs, postoperative patients who have had a general anesthetic are reminded to take deep breaths periodically so that adequate respiratory function can be restored.

Measurement of the blood pressure is the last one of the group of vital signs. The determination of blood pressure gives an indication of the effort that is being exerted by the heart and the condition of the arterial walls.[3] In patients who have suffered shock for any reason, the blood pressure will be low. This is particularly true of patients who have suffered extensive blood loss through injury or surgery. Elevation in blood pressure usually occurs as a result of pathology of the heart or blood vessels, but other illnesses can contribute to deviations in this direction.

When the blood pressure is observed, two readings are taken. The first is the systolic pressure or the amount of pressure exerted by the contraction of the ventricles. The other reading is the diastolic, or the amount of pressure existing when the ventricles are in the relaxed phase of the cardiac cycle. The range of blood pressure which generally is accepted as normal is from seventy to ninety, diastolic, and one hundred to one hundred thirty, systolic. The blood pressure reading is recorded as systolic/diastolic. Sometimes, the heart sound can be heard even as the mercury falls to zero, but a marked change may be detectable at

---

[3]Elinor Fuerst and LuVerne Wolff, *Fundamentals of Nursing* (Philadelphia: J. B. Lippincott Company, 1964), page 181.

some point. When this happens, it is recommended that the diastolic reading be recorded so that both the point of change in sound and zero are shown.

PAIN

For as long as man has been able to record his experiences, one problem that has been common to all men is that of pain.[4] The problem of pain, as yet, is not understood fully even though numerous research projects have been conducted and others are in process at the present time. The purposes of some research studies on pain are to determine the exact nature of the mechanism of pain and to develop ways in which relief can be afforded directly. When central nervous system depressants are given for the relief of pain, they do not attack the actual cause of the pain but cause the patient to be unaware of the discomfort. The fact that people experience pain is accepted as true, and when a patient says he has pain, he really is experiencing pain. Pain can arise as a result of many problems, and only the patient can describe and pinpoint the pain he is experiencing. No one can say for a patient just how severe his pain is or can determine whether he really has it. Therefore, it becomes necessary that a complaint of pain be respected and appropriate measures taken to relieve it. Until such time as the research findings reveal more about the mechanisms involved in pain and its relief, it is necessary to make the best of methods now available.

Upon looking at a patient, one cannot discern specifically how that patient feels. Pain has no external manifestation such as redness, swelling, or rash. However, the patient's facial expression and other behavior might give some clue as to the presence of discomfort. Behavior is not always an accurate indicator of the extent of pain, however. Different people have different capacities for pain tolerance and, while one patient may show outward signs of severe discomfort in the presence of minor pain, another may show almost no outward sign of discomfort in the presence of severe pain.[5] For this reason, the nurse must attempt to evaluate and interpret what she sees and hears in order to make a judgment about the real condition of the patient.

What, then, are the ways in which a nurse can determine if a patient has pain if he does not complain? Actually, there are several signals which should alert the nurse to this fact. If the patient is bedfast, he

---

[4]John Hunter, "The Mark of Pain," *American Journal of Nursing*, Vol. 61, No. 10, 1961, pages 96-99.

[5]M. A. Kaufman and D. E. Brown, "Pain Wears Many Faces," *American Journal of Nursing*, Vol. 61, No. 1, 1961, pages 48-51.

may reveal his discomfort through such behaviors as restlessness, withdrawal from the situation by trying to lie quietly or to sleep, changes in facial expression, or, if able and willing, by calling for help. The facial expression may be a signal even if the patient appears to be sleeping. He may be wearing a grimace which reveals the tension in his face.

Sometimes, patients will hesitate to call upon the nurse for help even though they have been instructed that they should feel free to do so. Without being aware of it, nurses frequently have such a businesslike manner and appear to be so coldly efficient that patients feel any interruption would be an inconvenience to the nurse. Therefore, nurses must try to work with an attitude of interest in and concern for their patients. This may be difficult when there are so many who need so much, but at least an effort in this direction will be appreciated by those who are suffering. Even when pain is inevitable, patients will be able to relax more if they know they can feel free to call for help when it is needed and that measures will be taken without delay to relieve the pain.

Whenever a patient experiences pain when he is ambulating or is in any type of motion, the considerate nurse will help the patient devise some plan for his activity that causes the least amount of discomfort and will see to it that any needed assistance is provided. It will be of great help to any patient who is experiencing pain if the nurse will communicate specifically to the other members of the nursing staff exactly what type of pain the patient has and what measures seem to afford the most relief. Patients grow very tired of having to repeat the same description and directions as often as new faces appear. With changes in staff occurring so rapidly, an almost continuous need for explanation by the patient is needed. It must be remembered, too, that pain is very tiring, and the patient who is experiencing pain will become fatigued easily.

Several adjectives have been used to describe the characteristics of pain. Some of them are sharp, penetrating, piercing, dull, aching, stabbing, crushing, intermittent, throbbing, and constant. It is the responsibility of the nurse to determine just what the nature of the pain is. Sometimes, it is difficult to get an exact description from the patient who should describe it in his own words, but this is essential. Suggesting adjectives may only confuse the patient with the result that contradictory statements may be made.

When the nurse reports a patient's complaint of pain to the physician, she should include in her report the duration as well as the intensity and location of the pain. She should include, also, a description of any medication given the patient and the length of time elapsed since the medication was administered. All of this information is essential for the physician to be able to prescribe the next move.

HEMORRHAGE

The sight of blood is usually disturbing enough to arouse concern since it is an established fact that blood is normally contained within the circulatory system, and the circulatory system is a closed system, with no external surface. Therefore, the presence of blood on the external surface of the body suggests that some kind of trauma has occurred to cause a disruption in the continuity of this closed system. When the nurse sees blood on a patient, her task is to determine the source and the amount of blood present. Only excessive bleeding is referred to as hemorrhage.

If the patient has had surgery, the first place to look would be the surgical incision. It is possible that a small vessel has not been ligated properly, thus permitting the escape of blood. It is also possible that some injury has occurred through moving or inadvertent disturbance of the dressings covering the wound. Whatever the cause, the extent of the bleeding should be determined, and if mild pressure does not stop the bleeding within a reasonable period, the surgeon or one of his assistants should be notified. Surgical correction may be necessary to protect the patient from extensive blood loss.

When blood appears on the external surface of the body in the absence of a surgical incision, the nurse must determine its source and extent. In the event of a laceration, mild pressure may be all that is needed to control the bleeding. It is important to establish whether a patient has fallen or bumped into a sharp object if there is no apparent cause for the bleeding. While it is unlikely that a patient would fall without the nurse being summoned either by the sound or by another patient, patients can fall unnoticed in bathrooms or hallways. In the event that a patient does fall, examination by the physician is imperative to determine whether injuries have occurred. When patients sustain lacerations, prompt and proper closure is necessary to promote healing, to prevent scarring, and to protect from infection.

If bleeding is occurring at the site of an area which has been scratched by the patient, the nurse should cleanse the wound thoroughly and protect it from further insult. Scratching is always a possibility if a patient has a rash or other irritation that is producing itching. Without even being aware that he is doing it, the patient can scratch himself until he causes considerable trauma. This may occur especially while the patient is sleeping. Also, the problem of scratching can be difficult to control in children. The child is aware only of the discomfort that he is experiencing, and he reacts almost instinctively to relieve it. Protection of the site can be afforded in part by cleansing and trimming the fingernails closely. Fingernails are potentially dangerous because of the warm moist area underneath them which serves as a well-protected spot for microorganisms.

Bleeding from internal sources poses a much greater problem for the nurse. In the first place, the site of the bleeding will not be nearly so detectable. However, in most cases of internal bleeding, there will be some outward, observable manifestation if the nurse is alert enough to see it. If the organ from which the bleeding is occurring has any communication with the exterior, blood may be present in the discharge or excreta from that organ. For this reason, all body discharges and excreta should be examined for the presence of blood. This does not mean necessarily that microscopic examinations should be made of every specimen, but that the nurse should become so alert to the characteristics of the various discharges and excreta that she would be able to detect the presence of blood at a glance. The first specimen that appears to contain blood should be reserved for inspection by the physician. Microscopic examination for occult blood may be ordered if bleeding is suspected in such small amounts that it is not readily detectable.

There are some medical diagnoses which should alert the nurse immediately to observe the patient for signs of bleeding. For example, even the tentative diagnosis of peptic or duodenal ulcer should suggest to the nurse that there is a possibility of bleeding. The blood would appear either in vomitus or in feces. Other diagnoses which suggest the possibility of gastrointestinal bleeding are esophageal varices, malignancies of the gastrointestinal tract, and hemorrhoids.

Because of the changes that occur in the blood as a result of the digestive process, it is important to note the color of the blood that is seen. Not all blood will appear as the natural, bright red that is so characteristic of blood. If it is fresh blood, that is, if it is coming from a source near the opening through which it is being expelled, it will be the characteristic bright red. If, however, it has occurred in the presence of digestive juices, the blood may have been partially digested, changing it to a dark, almost black color. Thus, when there is gradual bleeding in the stomach, the patient may vomit coffee-ground material which is caused by the digestive action upon the blood. If there is heavy bleeding such as in esophageal varices, the blood will probably be its usual bright red.

When blood is observed in the stool, again it may be either bright red or dark and tarry. The appearance of bright red blood in the stool means that the blood has come from a source which is below the site of digestion. The appearance of a black, tarry stool indicates that there is bleeding high enough in the digestive tract so that the blood is partially digested. Black, tarry stools are almost inevitable when patients have bleeding in the small intestine. When a nurse suspects that she is seeing this type of blood in the stool, she must be careful to ascertain that she is not being deceived by changes in the stool produced by certain foods and medications such as iron and green leafy vegetables. Also the ingestion of large quantities of red beets may cause the stool to have a red appearance.

Presence of blood in urine is readily identifiable unless it is present in a very minute quantity, which is detectable only upon microscopic examination. When there is considerable bleeding within the urinary tract, the urine will take on a pink or even bright red color. In the event of gross bleeding in the urinary tract, small clots may be present in the urine. This type of bleeding is usually accompanied by severe pain on urination. Observation of these signs requires the nurse to report the situation so that proper treatment can be initiated.

Presence of blood in the sputum can occur as a result of various respiratory disorders. The appearance of the blood may vary according to the problem which is causing it. One respiratory problem accompanied by blood in the sputum is pneumonia. When a patient has pneumonia, the color of the sputum will vary from a pinkish color to a rusty color as the disease progresses and the red blood cells break down. Diseases, such as malignancies and tuberculosis which are invasive, may produce erosion of the blood vessels within the lung tissue and frank, red blood, in varying quantities, may be expectorated.

When bleeding is occurring within body parts which have no external orifice, the nurse must observe for other signs. Perhaps the most valid indicator is the measurement of the blood pressure. While analysis of some characteristics of the blood pressure will require more skill and knowledge than the nurse may possess, measurement of the systolic and diastolic pressures are within the ability of the nurse. A graphic record of periodic measurements will provide a clear picture of what is happening within the patient's circulatory system, and the nurse need not wait for specific direction to initiate such a record when she observes a change in the patient's blood pressure. Even if the record is not necessary, it is better to have made and recorded frequent observations than to ignore changes which could be significant.

Along with changes in blood pressure, there are some other signals of internal bleeding to be observed. Whenever the nurse is observing any patient who may be susceptible to internal hemorrhage, she should be alerted if the patient becomes restless and seems apprehensive. These symptoms are often a prelude to hemorrhage. In response, the nurse should check the patient's pulse. Sometimes, the pulse will seem rather strong and bounding if hemorrhage has not occurred yet. If this is found to be the case, the nurse should check the pulse periodically so that she can detect quickly any change in its characteristics. A weak and rapid pulse is a signal that there is a problem at hand. In some cases, the adjective thready is used to describe the pulse of a patient who is in shock. While there are many causes for shock, the sudden loss of blood is the one with which this discussion is concerned. A thready pulse can be identified by its characteristic of seeming to run along in a continuous stream as a thread which has slightly detectable knots at periodic intervals. Such a pulse means that the heart is contracting more rapidly in an attempt to compensate for the blood loss that is occurring. As the heart works so much harder, it becomes fatigued and its contractions are weaker.

Another change in the patient who is bleeding internally will be in his skin color. The skin will lose its normal pinkish tone and take on a pale and sometimes almost ashen-gray appearance. The lips and nailbeds may appear to be bluish or white, and if pressed gently, the usual prompt return of color is not seen. Hands and feet may seem cold, also.

Before any of these signs are permitted to continue for any appreciable length of time, the physician should be notified so that treatments to control the bleeding and to support the overall condition of the patient may be initiated. Early attention may preclude the necessity for surgical intervention. However, this sometimes is the only means to bring about correction of the problem.

Bleeding from any of the body orifices is a signal of the existence of a problem except, of course, in the case of normal menstruation. It, therefore, becomes the responsibility of the nurse to pay particular attention to the site of the bleeding and to notify the physician if the bleeding continues for any appreciable length of time. One of the most common sites of bleeding is from the nose. When epistaxis does occur, the patient should be instructed to rest quietly, applying mild pressure with tissues. In order to determine the amount of blood lost, it is helpful if the tissues are reserved in a suitable receptacle until they are seen by the physician. Epistaxis can reflect and pose serious problems and, for this reason, the patient should receive medical attention.

Regardless of the source or extent of any bleeding, the appearance of blood deserves immediate attention so that appropriate measures can be taken to prevent complications.

EDEMA

Edema is an accumulation of fluid in the extracellular spaces causing the area to increase in size. It can occur in any part of the body and is easily discernible over any visible body part. It is a sign of such disorders as trauma, allergic inflammatory reaction, circulatory impairment, and dysfunction of the renal and endocrine systems. When mild pressure is applied to the edematous part with the fingers and the imprint of the fingers remains as fluid is pushed into the surrounding extracellular spaces, it is described as pitting edema. The length of time required for these indentations to refill is significant.

In the presence of kidney disease, edema may be observed in several parts of the body such as in the feet and ankles, the fingers, and around the eyes. The problem of ankle edema is magnified by the fact that the feet are usually in a dependent position.

In some types of heart disease which impair the ability of the heart to pump blood into the arterial system of the remainder of the body as rapidly as it is pumping blood into the pulmonary artery, the blood pools in the lungs with the consequent development of pulmonary edema. The development of this condition presents several signals which are recognizable by the nurse: shortness of breath, noisy respirations and coughing which is productive of frothy, blood-tinged sputum. Any of these signals should alert the nurse to seek the aid of a physician immediately as pulmonary edema is generally considered to be a medical emergency.

When patients have generalized edema involving the extremities, it is important to examine the sacral area for the presence of edema. Because edema renders the skin more vulnerable to injury, meticulous attention is essential to prevent the breakdown of the skin and decubitus formation.

Another site at which edema sometimes occurs is within the cranium. Edema occurring within the cranium can produce serious increase in the intracranial pressure. If it continues uncontrolled, the effects may be damaging to the vital centers and can ultimately produce cessation of their ability to maintain life.

When edema occurs as a manifestation of an allergic reaction, the area which comes in contact with the allergen is the site most affected. While some reactions are mild, others are severe and require emergency treatment. The administration of antihistamines may be ordered by the physician to help decrease the allergic reaction and, consequently, the edema.

COUGH

Coughing is the body's means of expelling from the respiratory tree any secretions or irritating substances which might be injurious if retained. If a patient is unable to cough, collections of mucus can cause obstruction in the air passageways, and these obstructions can increase the danger of pulmonary infections. Obstruction also interferes with the body's ability to carry on the essential respiratory function of obtaining the oxygen needed for metabolism and the excreting of carbon dioxide and water, the waste products of metabolism.

Whenever a nurse hears a patient cough, she should listen carefully to determine whether it is a dry, hacking cough or a productive cough. The patient should be provided with an adequate supply of tissues to receive material expectorated and a disposable container to receive these tissues. Paper bags or cartons attached to the bed or bedside cabinet serve as effective receptacles. These receptacles should be replaced as often as necessary so that the danger of spread of infection is reduced.

The nurse should observe also the characteristics of the sputum. The mucus which is secreted normally to serve as a lubricant for the mucous membrane is a clear and odorless liquid. In the presence of infection, the sputum may contain pus which would change its color and consistency. If bleeding is occurring, the sputum may appear to be red-tinged or perhaps rusty as in the progress of pneumonia.

Patients should be taught to protect others from their coughs by covering their mouths properly. Many infections are spread by droplets, and the distance that droplets may be carried by a vigorous cough is much greater than one might suspect. The nurse can protect herself from the cough of her patient by instructing him to turn his head away from her.

In some cases, patients require treatments which are directed toward loosening the secretions to be removed by coughing. Instruction is necessary to enable the patient to cough effectively. In the event of a dry, hacking cough, the therapy may be medication to suppress the cough. If such is the case, the nurse must observe for its effectiveness and may administer additional doses as necessary.

Occasional coughing may be quite normal and of no serious import, but any patient with a persistent cough should be observed carefully and should be managed according to the directions of the physician.

NAUSEA AND VOMITING

Nausea is a subjective symptom which occurs in response to both physical and psychological stimuli. Some examples of stimuli which can produce it are trauma, foods which are spoiled, medications, motion, and emotional upsets. Nausea may or may not be accompanied by vomiting. When it occurs alone, the person feels as if he will vomit, and any measures that can be taken to decrease this sensation will be received most gratefully by the patient. It is known that motion tends to increase nausea and, therefore, the patient should be encouraged to lie as quietly as possible. Any turning that must be done should be done slowly and without unnecessary motion. Antiemetics, if ordered by the physician, can be given also. Some patients can be helped by breathing deeply through the mouth.

When vomiting accompanies nausea, the stomach empties itself of the irritating contents by means of violent contraction of the muscles in the stomach wall. Sometimes, the irritation is severe enough that these contractions continue after the stomach has been emptied of its contents. Such retching can be very painful for the patient. Even the contraction of the stomach and abdominal muscles which occurs during vomiting can cause enough soreness to produce considerable discomfort.

When vomiting occurs, the nurse should observe whether it is preceded and accompanied by retching or if it just happens suddenly without warning. Sudden, vigorous vomiting is known as projectile vomiting, and it occurs as a response to stimuli in the central nervous system. Projectile vomiting is characterized by the force with which the vomitus is emitted as well as by the absence of retching. It is seen frequently in patients with cerebral pathology which causes increased intracranial pressure.

Prolonged vomiting can cause dehydration and serious electrolyte imbalance. Therefore, patients who have persistent nausea and vomiting are given parenteral fluid therapy to maintain adequate hydration and electrolyte levels. Food and fluids may not be given by mouth until the problem which is producing the nausea and vomiting has been solved.

Appropriate receptacles should be kept within easy reach of the patient who is suffering from nausea and vomiting. The nurse should observe the amount and characteristics of all vomitus. Specimens are reserved for inspection by the physican when unusual observations are made.

Care should be taken to remove vomitus and any soiled clothing or linens from the patient's bedside. Vomitus produces an odor which is offensive to the patient and to those around him. The patient should be provided with water or mouthwash, if desired, to rinse his mouth to remove the unpleasant taste caused by the vomitus.

ABDOMINAL DISTENTION

Distention of the abdomen can occur as a result of several medical disorders, and the nurse should be alert to the development of it. Patients who have had abdominal surgery are subject to this problem if there is any delay in the reestablishment of peristalsis. Normally, when the abdominal muscles are relaxed as they are when a person lies on his back, the abdomen is soft, but with the accumulation of gas or fluid either in the intestines or in the peritoneal cavity, the abdominal wall becomes stretched and taut. The abdomen of patients who have ascites, which is the collection of fluid in the abdominal cavity, may become so distended that changes occur in the external appearance of the abdomen. The umbilicus may protrude, and the skin over the abdomen may take on a thin, glossy appearance.

When abdominal distention occurs as a result of the absence of peristalsis, the physician will prescribe treatment directed toward the reestablishment of peristalsis. The nurse will need to observe the patient for the presence of flatulence. Sometimes, the insertion of a rectal tube is prescribed to aid in the release of flatulence. Whenever a rectal tube is inserted, the nurse must help evaluate its effectiveness by her observation.

Another problem which contributes to abdominal distention is the inability of a patient to void. The bladder wall has considerable elasticity to enable it to contain a larger quantity of urine than the usual 200 to 400 c.c. required to provide the stimulus to empty the bladder. As the amount of urine increases, the bladder becomes so distended that its outline becomes palpable and sometimes even visible above the symphysis pubis. This situation causes discomfort to the patient and poses a hazard to the well-being of the patient in that such distention can damage the cells in the bladder wall sufficiently to produce the loss of muscle tone. Postoperative patients, patients with back injuries, and patients who have received large amounts of depressant drugs should be observed closely for the problem of bladder distention.

NUMBNESS

Numbness is a symptom which is perceptible only to the patient. It may occur in the presence of neurological problems or circulatory problems. Regardless of its cause, it is the loss of sensation over a part. Because it means that there is a loss of sensory perception, there are certain considerations which must be kept in mind to safeguard the patient. First, patients who have numbness over their extremities could be burned easily if they were to come into contact with a hot object. Therefore, the use of any heating devices such as hot water bottles or heating pads is contraindicated. Consider, for example, a patient with numbness due to inadequate circulation to a part. Not only would the person be injured, but the healing process would be hindered by the lack of circulation to bring nutrients to the part. As a result, what appeared to be a minor injury might develop into a complicated problem which requires prolonged and meticulous management.

Another consideration for which the nurse must be on guard in the case of patients with this problem is the protection of the part from any objects or positions which could cause injury to the part. If the patient has lost sensation of a part, he could sustain injury without being aware of it. The nurse should test the affected part periodically to determine whether the area of numbness is changing in any way.

DISCOLORATIONS OF SKIN

Many kinds of skin discoloration can be seen as signs of injury or disease. Even the redness which occurs as a result of sunburn should be considered a discoloration because it is, in fact, the result of a burn. Other discolorations may result from bruising the tissue, capillary bleeding, or changes in pigmentation.

The capillary bleeding which appears as red or reddish blue pinpoint spots, known as petechiae, accompanies various blood dyscrasias. It can be seen first in areas which are free of hair such as in the bend of the elbow. Another type of discoloration which accompanies blood dyscrasias is the spotted discoloration known as purpura. The areas of discoloration which occur as bruises or injury are called ecchymosis. When a part appears to be blanched, it is described as ischemic or suffering from inadequate blood supply. Cyanosis is another word used to describe a problem with circulation. Cyanosis is a bluish discoloration which results from an inadequate supply of oxygen to a part. There may be circulation, but the red blood cells are not carrying the necessary oxygen.

Changes in the amount of pigmentation can be brought about by exposure to the ultraviolet rays of the sun or by certain endocrine disorders. Changes which develop because of endocrine disorders usually appear over only parts of the body and, when they are seen, the nurse should be tactful in any attention she calls to them. Women, particularly, may feel very self-conscious about their presence.

ITCHING

Itching is an example of a subjective symptom in that only the patient can feel or experience this problem. Its cause, however, is frequently visible to the examiner, and the observation of a patient scratching any part of his anatomy should serve as a summons to the nurse to learn the cause. Itching is often observed in patients who are jaundiced as a result of liver disease. Rashes or irritating bed clothes can be responsible for itching also. Whatever the cause, the nurse should take the palliative measures at her disposal to relieve the itching and prevent further injury to the skin.

Rashes and urticaria should be reported to the physician who will decide what has produced these reactions and what to do about them. Medications are common causes of such reactions. If such is the case, the causative factor is eliminated, and frequently an antihistamine agent is ordered to give the patient fairly rapid relief.

HICCOUGHS

Hiccoughing is caused by spasmodic contractions of the diaphragm which is stimulated by the phrenic nerve. While they may be short-lived and produce no harmful effects in the majority of patients, hiccoughs can cause considerable discomfort in postoperative patients and in anyone in whom they persist for any appreciable length of time. Many remedies have been tried, and while some patients are relieved by them, others continue to suffer. Whenever a nurse observes that a patient has hiccoughs that persist, she should seek the advice of the attending physician to attempt to effect relief.

ERUCTATION

The act of belching, or eructation, is produced by the escape of gas from the stomach. This may occur, to a minimal extent, in a person who enjoys good health. Excessive eructation may occur in the presence of certain gastrointestinal or liver dysfunctions. Observation and accurate reporting of the occurrence of eructation is important so that proper treatment can be instituted.

DRAINAGE AND DISCHARGES

There are many instances when a nurse is called upon to observe and describe the drainage or discharge from a wound or body orifice. The word discharge is usually used to refer to material excreted through a normal body orifice, whereas drainage is usually used to mean the material which escapes from a wound.

There are as many types of body discharges as there are orifices. The normal discharge from the eyes is the clear, watery liquid which is produced by the lacrimal glands and which serves as a lubricant for the eyes. In crying, there is excessive secretion of this fliud to form tears. The presence of tearing in the absence of crying and any other type of discharge such as bleeding or purulent material should be noted and reported.

The normal discharge from the ear is an amber, waxy substance called cerumen. It, also, is a lubricant and cleansing agent and should be removed only as it enters the outer part of the ear. The presence of a very dark, hardened wax may be an indication of a collection of hardened wax in the ear canal. Such a collection can cause sufficient obstruction to interfere with the hearing of the patient. Irrigation may be necessary to remove collections of cerumen.

Wherever a body orifice is lined with mucous membrane, as is the nose, one can expect to see some discharge of the clear, mucus secretion. In the presence of upper respiratory infections, the amount of nasal discharge will be increased markedly, and its appearance will change to become purulent or possibly blood tinged.

Vaginal discharges at times other than during menses are usually minimal in quantity. In the presence of infection in the vaginal canal, there may be large amounts of discharge which may or may not be purulent and which may be characterized by an offensive odor.

Discharge from the anus is extremely rare except with the due process of defecation. Any additional discharge would warrant the attention of the physician. The characteristics to be observed concerning the products of elimination are discussd in Chapter 2.

Discharge from the urethra may be seen in the presence of infections. A purulent discharge is seen in the presence of infection, and the nurse must exercise aseptic technique to insure her own protection from contamination. Since urine is a normal product of excretion, it is not considered to be an unusual discharge. However, when a patient has an indwelling catheter in place, the urine is referred to as urinary drainage. Characteristics of urine to be observed are described in Chapter 2.

Drainage which appears at the site of a wound, surgical or traumatic, should always be examined for characteristics and amount. When the drainage is clear to yellowish, it is described as serous meaning that its chief component is serum. This is the type of fluid that appears in a blister resulting from second degree burns. If the discharge contains serum which is blood tinged, it is called serosanguineous. Sanguineous drainage is composed chiefly of blood.

The appearance of sanguineous drainage calls for close observation and appropriate measures to prevent extensive blood loss. When drainage appears to be excessive, steps should be initiated to have the wound examined by the physician who will determine the subsequent course of action.

Drainage collecting on dressings may produce offensive odors if the dressings are not changed periodically. Drainage resulting from infected wounds is much more noxious than the serous drainage which may occur normally. Therefore, the detection of a strong, foul odor about a patient with a wound warrants prompt attention.

Disposal of soiled dressings should be handled in such a way that all patients and personnel are protected. Disposable gloves can be used to change contaminated dressings, and then the gloves and dressings should be wrapped in a piece of paper or placed in a paper bag before being deposited in a waste can. The waste can should have a tight fitting lid so that disease carrying insects cannot get to these dressings. The practice of discarding dressings in waste baskets is to be abhorred regardless of whether the dressing is wet or dry. A nurse observing any one disposing of a dressing in such a way is obligated to inform that person of appropriate disposal methods and to assist with proper disposition. Proper handling is essential for the safety of personnel and patients.

PERSPIRATION

Perspiration represents one of the routes of excretion of body wastes. Also, the evaporation of perspiration produces a cooling effect and enables man to endure higher atmospheric temperatures. A certain amount of perspiration is normal and essential. However, in the presence of some disease conditions, the patient perspires more than usual. For example, following the crisis of fever, the patient may perspire quite profusely. Excessive perspiration of this sort is known as diaphoresis. Diaphoresis can occur in the presence of other maladies, too, or just when a person who is weak from illness or surgery attempts to sit or stand.

Whenever diaphoresis occurs, the nurse should observe the extent of the patient's body that appears to be involved. She should provide dry clothing and bed linens as often as necessary. Although it can provide only a rough estimate, one way of describing the amount of perspiration is by the frequency with which clothing and linen changes are needed and the degree of saturation at the time of change.

Care should be taken to prevent exposure of the patient to drafts which may cause chilling. Exposure by itself does not cause colds to develop, but it can help to lower the body resistance to organisms that may be present and, hence, increase the chances of the development of a respiratory infection. Dampness can cause muscle and joint discomfort, also. So, for the comfort of the patient, the nurse must try to keep his clothing and bedding dry.

CHILLS

Chills usually are associated with fever in that the chill occurs in response to the body's need for an increase in temperature. Realizing that fever is a defense mchanism, one can understand that it is not completely bad. The complications arise when the temperature rises so high that brain tissue is affected. When a chill does occur, the patient may experience violent, uncontrollable shaking. The nurse should add blankets and, unless contraindicated, a covered hot water bottle applied to the feet will help the patient to feel warm again and cause the shaking to cease. The length and severity of a chill should be noted, and the patient's temperature should be taken as soon as the chill is over. It can be expected that the temperature will be elevated. It is not a good idea to take the temperature orally during a chill as the danger of breaking the thermometer is increased by the shaking.

DIZZINESS

Dizziness is an example of a subjective symptom. No one but the patient really knows exactly what he experiences. Dizziness can occur with a variety of health problems ranging from weakness resulting from mild upsets to serious problems involving the various body systems, and whenever it occurs, it deserves attention. Dizziness may be a forerunner of syncope, and the nurse must respect a patient's complaint of this problem and should take precautionary measures to insure safety. The sudden onset of dizziness may be an indication of some serious circulatory or neurological disorder, and for this reason, it should be brought to the attention of the physician.

Because of the possibility of dizziness occurring following periods of bedrest or surgical treatment, the nurse is advised to take precautionary measures in assisting these patients. In addition to determining the rate and quality of the pulse, the nurse is advised to assist the patient to the upright position gradually. The patient should be helped to sit long enough to feel steady in that position before he attempts to stand. A cautious nurse will have a chair handy, and if she suspects that there is a likelihood of the occurrence of dizziness, she will seek aid before attempting to get the patient out of bed.

SUMMARY

Discussion in this chapter has centered around specific observations of symptoms manifested by people who are ill. In order to give intelligent nursing care, the nurse must have a background of knowledge of symptoms to be observed and their significance. Through constant and accurate observation, the alert nurse can contribute a great deal to the care and well-being of her patients.

BIBLIOGRAPHY

CHAFFEE, ELLEN E., and GREISHEIMER, ESTHER M., *Basic Physiology and Anatomy.* Philadelphia: J. B. Lippincott Company, 1964.

FUERST, ELINOR V., and WOLFF, LUVERNE, *Fundamentals of Nursing.* Philadelphia: J. B. Lippincott Company, 1964.

HOPPS, HOWARD C., *Principles of Pathology.* New York: Appleton-Century-Crofts, Inc., 1964.

HUNTER, JOHN, "The Mark of Pain," *American Journal of Nursing,* Vol. 61, No. 10, 1961, pp. 96-99.

KAUFMANN, MARGARET A., and BROWN, DOROTHY E., "Pain Wears Many Faces," *American Journal of Nursing,* Vol. 61, No. 1, 1961, pp. 48-51.

KRUG, ELSIE E., *Pharmacology in Nursing,* 9th ed. St. Louis: The C. V. Mosby Company, 1963.

MACBRYDE, CYRIL, editor, *Signs and Symptoms.* Philadelphia: J. B. Lippincott Company, 1964.

MATHENEY, RUTH V., and others, *Fundamentals of Patient-Centered Nursing.* St. Louis: The C. V. Mosby Company, 1964.

"Recognizing Early Signs of Internal Hemorrhage," *American Journal of Nursing,* Vol. 65, No. 12, 1965, pp. 119-138.

SHAFER, KATHLEEN, and others, *Medical-Surgical Nursing,* 3rd ed. St. Louis: The C. V. Mosby Company, 1964.

SMITH, DOROTHY W., and GIPS, CLAUDIA D., *Care of the Adult Patient,* 2nd ed. Philadelphia: J. B. Lippincott Company, 1966.

Chapter _____ 4

Observations Related
to Nursing Activities

As she attends to the needs of the patient, the nurse has unique opportunities to observe the patient. The observations that she makes may
be of purely physical factors, or they may be related to the psychological
state or behavior of the patient. Awareness that one is being observed
tends to create an unnatural situation, but the nurse learns to observe
the patient in a less obvious or overt manner. The discussion in this
chapter suggests ways in which the nurse can utilize opportunities for
observation in typical situations.

ADMITTING THE PATIENT

When a patient enters the hospital, there are several observations
which the nurse must make in order to determine just how much assistance will be required by him.[1] There is usually a standard admission
procedure which requires information about the problem that has
brought about the need for hospitalization, the recording of the vital
signs, and a notation about the means by which the patient arrived on
the unit. Also, the nurse is expected to make a note of any unusual
observations which she may make, such as evidence of any injury to
the skin or edema of any part of the body. During this time, it would
be wise for the nurse to provide as much privacy for the patient as
possible, remembering that both men and women are modest and their
rights must be respected courteously.

While the inspection made by the nurse is not as detailed as the
physical examination by the physician, there are several important ob-

---

[1]Fuerst and Wolff, *op. cit.*, page 135.

servations regarding the general condition of the patient. As she takes his vital signs, the nurse can observe the condition of skin and the hair to ascertain their general state. Rarely are pediculi found, but when they are, early attention is required to prevent their spread. The nurse must use discretion as she assists the patient and must avoid embarrassing him. Sometimes, patients bring such vermin as bedbugs to the hospital in their clothing, and the nurse must be alert to this possibility as she assists the patient in putting away his belongings. Any evidence of insect bites on the patient should be noted for inspection by the physician. The use of good judgment will enable the nurse to decide which patients require this type of scrutiny.

The presence of any open skin lesions should be called to the attention of the physician who will determine their cause and recommend treatment. Any drainage from such wounds should be handled carefully to avoid contamination as the nurse observes its characteristics and disposes of it, regardless of its source.

As the nurse assists the patient in getting himself settled comfortably, she can make some assessment of the general physical strength of the patient. Does he seem to fatigue easily? Is he unable to walk without support? Is he lethargic and listless? The sick person must not be expected to be as cheerful and exuberant as the person who is in a state of good health. The facial expression reveals quite a lot about a person, and for this reason, it should be observed closely.

Observable handicaps should be noted so that the patient can receive whatever assistance is needed without being subjected to repeated questioning about the handicaps. Blindness is usually a rather obvious handicap but impaired vision may not be. If the patient has an artificial eye, provision should be made for its care. Another common problem is deafness. Regardless of whether the patient has a hearing aid, the problem should be noted with the suggestion that all personnel speak slowly and distinctly.

Examples of other types of handicaps the patient may have include problems with speech, the use of the hands or arms, locomotion, and ability to control elimination. Speech defects can be embarrassing and frustrating to patients, and for this reason, special effort should be made to listen carefully when the patient speaks to reduce the need for repetition. If a patient has limited use of his hands and arms, provisions should be made to afford as much convenience as possible to enable the patient to do as much as he can for himself. Necessary assistance should be offered tactfully. Any difficulty in the ability to move about should be noted, and provision should be made for whatever assistance is needed. Patients who are permitted to walk but who have difficulty doing so should be assigned a unit which is convenient to toilet facilities.

All patients whose condition permits should be oriented to the environment of the hospital unit, including introduction to their neighbors. The nurse makes certain that there is a functioning call bell or other signaling device within easy reach of the patient. She should ascertain whether the patient is able to participate in some diversional activity. If he is, he should be guided to the facilities available and should be encouraged to do as much as his condition permits. Patients should not be permitted to become overly fatigued regardless of their interests in diversion.

Patients are bathed on admission only when their condition demands it. Occasionally, patients whose hygiene demands immediate attention can be examined more adequately by the physician if a bath is given first. This is particularly true of those whose work requires them to become quite soiled or people whose ability to attend to their own hygiene is limited.

Although the nurse should observe all of the foregoing characteristics of patients, only those observations which seem unusual or pertinent need to be reported and recorded. Otherwise, nurse's notes would become so voluminous that their worth would be curtailed.

CONVERSATIONS WITH PATIENTS

Conversations with patients should be meaningful. A "gift of gab" is not enough when a nurse meets and talks with a new patient. Congeniality helps to put the patient at ease, but it is not enough when a patient is trying to discuss his illness. The patient is concerned primarily with his health problem and is much more interested in getting well than in discussing such irrelevant subjects as the weather or the problems of the nurse. It has happened that nurses have been so preoccupied with their own thoughts that they have not permitted the patient to express his concerns. Many books have been written on interviewing techniques, and it is not the purpose here to delve into a long dissertation on the skill of interviewing. However, there is one aspect of interviewing that is basic to observation, and that is the art of listening. Did you ever try to sit and listen to someone else talk for five minutes without expressing any of your own opinions or making any other verbal response? All too often, because a person is so concerned with the idea that he wishes to express, he misses entirely the point that someone else is trying to make. If two people involved in a conversation would really listen to what the other is saying before interrupting with a response that might cut off further expression, they might find that not only is the conversation more satisfying but interpersonal relations would be improved greatly.

One of the most commonly used and least meant greetings is, "How are you?" Unfortunately, the use of this question has become so mechanical that, for the most part, no one wants to know how you really are. But, assuming that its use is well intended, did you ever stop to think how many people greet a patient with this question? He is expected to respond in the same way that everyone else does with a "Fine, thank you," or, "Feeling better, thank you." But suppose that he is not feeling fine or even any better, but worse. Will the person asking the question take the time to find out just how the patient is feeling? Because the answer is ignored so frequently, patients tire of trying to answer the question and either ignore it or just say, "Fine." With a little thought, anyone would know that the patient is not fine or he would not be in the hospital. Unfortunately for the patient, people usually accept his response of "Fine," and that is as far as it goes.

Instead of approaching patients with this cliché, the nurse should concentrate upon the patient and should ask questions that are more specific so that she can learn how the patient really is. Conversation must focus upon the problems of the patient if the nurse is to ascertain just what help he needs from her. The nurse should avoid introducing problems that are her own. This is not to say that there is never a time for a casual conversation between a nurse and a patient, but the art is in finding the appropriate time. It is to be expected that patients will have varied interests, and as their condition improves, they will be able to think of something besides their immediate health problems.

Learning to listen is a difficult task, especially for the beginner in nursing. The beginner is so involved, and rightly so, with her own new experiences that she is unable to reach beyond herself until she has developed some confidence in at least a few nursing activities. The most natural thing to do seems to be to reply to comments without stopping to analyze the real meaning of a comment. There is a need for nurses to know how people express themselves so that even a subtle request for someone to listen will be recognized.

Casual listening to a conversation is not enough for the nurse. Full attention with an open mind is essential for the nurse to hear what the patient is saying. In a brief speech of greeting to a new class of students, a director of a school of nursing stated that, of all the skills the nurse must develop, listening is one of the most valuable. Actually, listening is a part of observation. When combined with what is actually seen, those things heard often enable the nurse to detect problems pertinent to the well-being of the patient and to the treatment of his medical problem. Through continuity of care, a close relationship can develop between the nurse and patient, thereby enabling the patient to express problems that would never be recognized in a more intermittent or casual relationship. To illustrate the value of listening, the following patient situation is offered.

When Mrs. N first complained of itching, she was examined and was found to have a rash over her arms, legs, and body. Believing the rash to be an allergic reaction to a medication she had been receiving, the physician discontinued the order for the drug and prescribed an antihistamine. The rash persisted in spite of this treatment. As Nurse A worked with Mrs. N, she noted that Mrs. N appeared to be quite restless. From her conversation with Mrs. N, Nurse A concluded that Mrs. N was apprehensive about her medical problem and hospitalization. Eventually, Mrs. N told Nurse A that she had been considered a "worrier" for quite a long time.

As Nurse A reflected upon the situation, she recalled the various events which preceded the present situation. First, there was the onset of the rash, then the ineffectiveness of the medications, the restlessness of the patient, and the frequent periods of wondering about the activities and care of her children. Nurse A began to wonder if there may be another basis for the rash. She discussed all of these observations with the physician who agreed that, indeed, there were other factors involved. Attention was then focused upon helping Mrs. N work out solutions to some of the problems which she was having at home. Within a few days, the rash had disappeared and Mrs. N was showing signs of recovery from the medical problem which was the cause of her hospitalization.

Had this nurse ignored the comments of the patient, Mrs. N's rash might have been unrelieved for a much longer period, and her hospitalization would have been prolonged.

Consider another hypothetical situation in which a patient who has diabetes arrives at the emergency room with a very high blood sugar. From the many outward signs, the physician can establish that the patient is in need of medical attention and will proceed with the appropriate management. Because of his fear of punishment for not following instructions regarding his diet, the patient may choose not to tell anyone that he consumed a large portion of his favorite dessert which he just could not resist. Meanwhile, the diagnostic tests are ordered and everyone works diligently to discover the cause of his imbalance. To him, the physicians and nurses represent authority, and only an attitude of acceptance and non-punitive concern will encourage the patient to admit his action.

During conversations with the patient, the nurse might observe that certain topics seem to bother him. It might be his wife, his work, his family, or some other subject. For example, a nurse who was working with a middle-aged man who had suffered a myocardial infarction realized that this man seemed to become quite tense at the mention of his home situation. Suspecting that there must be a problem in the home, the nurse made it a point to be present when the patient's wife made her next visit. When the patient introduced the nurse to his wife, the wife greeted her warmly and appeared to be pleased to know who was responsible for the care of her husband. The nurse was able to detect the tension that existed between the patient and his wife throughout the visit. Subsequently, the nurse ascertained that there was a problem which the patient wished to discuss with his physician but had not done so, thinking that it might be irrelevant. At the encouragement of the nurse, the patient agreed to discuss the matter with the physician on his next visit. As a result, the patient received the assistance that he needed. Had the nurse ignored his reactions during their conversations, the patient could have recovered from his illness and been discharged to a situation that might have continued to disturb him and his family.

The question of confidentiality arises when it becomes necessary to report information gained through conversation. It must be recognized that conversations between nurse and physician about patients are purposeful and are considered confidential. Nurses must share pertinent information with the physician for the sake of the patient. On rare occasions, a patient may ask that the nurse not discuss what he has said with his physician. When such a request is made, the nurse should attempt to discover the basis for such a request. It is possible that the patient fears that he may hear the worst about his condition or that he may be scolded or even penalized for something which he considers a wrongdoing. If a patient makes this request prior to discussing a problem, the nurse should avoid promising that she will not relate the information to the physician. The information may be vital to the patient's welfare. On the other hand, it may be insignificant with no need for further transmission. When the nurse assures the patient that whatever she discusses with the physician is held in confidence, the patient can decide what he wishes to discuss further. Once the threat is removed, the patient will be likely to seek the help of the nurse. The very fact that he has asked to talk about the problem is evidence that it is bothering him sufficiently to deserve attention. But the decision must come from the patient with no coercion on the part of the nurse.

Conversations can be utilized for teaching, also. Some patient teaching takes place in formal teacher-learner situations, but much of it is done informally as the nurse administers care to the patient. Bath time, for example, provides an excellent opportunity for the nurse to reinforce learning by answering questions that may have arisen since the formal teaching occurred. This is a time, too, when the nurse can demonstrate to the patient the kind of care that the patient may need and later can allow the patient to take care of his own needs, with or without assistance. During this time, she may learn too that a patient has some poor health habits which need to be corrected through understanding.

Observation can be a starting point for meaningful and beneficial conversations with the patient. As in any teaching, evaluation of the learning should be made, and it is the nurse who can determine whether the teaching by the medical or nursing personnel has been effective.

BATHING THE PATIENT

Bath time for the bedfast patient affords the nurse a better opportunity than any other period during the day to observe thoroughly the overall condition of the patient.[2] More time is spent administering this care than in any other one nursing activity. Bath time provides an opportunity to observe any physical changes and to evaluate the patient's response to activity.

Observations to be made during a bath include skin changes such as presence of a rash, discoloration, edema, physical malformations, and any other unusual characteristics. The nurse should take advantage of this opportunity to check the progress in healing of any wounds that may be present. Because of the hazard of development of skin breakdown resulting from constant pressure or friction, the nurse should give particular attention to the bony prominences including elbows, heels, ankles, hips, sacral area, and the area over the scapulae.

Condition of the hair should be observed, also. In the presence of some disease conditions, the hair loses its luster and becomes difficult to manage because of excessive dryness or oiliness. The general hygiene of the hair is important, too, and though the occurrence of pediculi is fairly uncommon, the nurse should observe for evidence of these vermin.

As soon as patients are past the stage of their illness in which they are almost totally preoccupied with their physical discomforts, they will indicate an interest in appearance. The nurse should offer assistance with make-up as soon as a woman appears ready for it or encourage the male patient to shave if he is able. If the male patient is unable to

---

2*Ibid.*, page 290.

shave himself, the nurse or someone else should do this for him. Actually, realizing that one does present a well-groomed appearance provides a boost in morale to many people; the time required to help with these aspects of care is minimal when compared with the benefits derived.

Other aspects of general hygiene that may be observed at bath time are general cleanliness of all parts of the body, the presence of body odors, and nails that need attention. This is not to say that the nurse must force the patient to be as fastidious about hygiene as she may be, but she can at least make these observations which will help her to identify needs for health teaching. It is known that cleanliness does reduce the dangers of infections. The offensiveness of body odors causes a person to be rejected by others, and regardless of the outward expressions of the lack of concern, the nature of the human being requires that he be accepted by others. Tactful assistance with this problem can mean a great deal to the patient who, in all innocence, may not realize the basis for such a problem. A simple means of offering such help is to ask if he would like to apply some deodorant when the bath has been completed.

Oral hygiene is another important aspect of the overall physical care of patients. Poor dentition characterized by the presence of caries can provide a focus for persistent low-grade infections which serve as a continual health hazard to the patient. When patients are unable to assume responsibility for their own oral hygiene, the nurse should assume this responsibility for them. Careful attention to the cleanliness of the mouth of dehydrated patients can prevent the formation of sordes and subsequent infection.

Bath time offers the nurse an opportunity to observe the general physical state of a patient. She can determine how much strength the patient seems to have and, when he is permitted, can encourage him to participate in his care. In so doing, the nurse can detect weakness of any particular part of the body. She also can estimate more accurately the amount of exercise that the patient can perform without undue fatigue. Nurses are encouraged to help maintain muscle tone and joint function through the use of range of motion exercises. No force should be exerted to exaggerate the usual function of the part. The application of such force should be carried out only by the physical therapist and under medical supervision.

As the nurse assists the patient with his bath, she can use the opportunity for conversation to many advantages. First, she can ascertain the general frame of mind or mood of the patient. Mood is not so important as mood per se, but it may reflect the concern or worry that a patient is feeling about his illness. If there are problems which are interfering with his ability to relax and rest, attention should be given to them. The value of conversation as a guide to problems of the patient is discussed in more detail in the previous section of this chapter.

Although it may be desirable for patients to have their attention directed toward the more positive aspects of their situation, there may be instances when an outburst of anger or crying may be necessary to relieve tension that has been building. Any such outburst should be recognized for what it is and should be treated respectfully rather than ignored or taken as a personal affront. It must be remembered that the very loss of ability to bathe oneself constitutes an insult to the ego of the individual, and regardless of the situation, the nurse must work with an attitude of compassion which enables her to offer the kind of encouragement that is needed by the sick.

PREVENTING DECUBITI

Prevention of decubitus ulcers presents a challenging nursing problem. It has been said that decubiti occur as a direct result of inadequate nursing care. Even though it is known now that the nutritional state of the patient contributes to this problem, the importance of meticulous nursing care cannot be minimized. With a working knowledge of predisposing conditions and preventive measures, the nurse will be able to identify patients who may be prone to the development of decubiti, and she can begin early in the patient's hospital stay to administer the kind of care that will prevent this development or at least will minimize the problem.

The importance of the nutritional state of the patient is a key factor in determining which patients may be susceptible to the development of decubiti. Questions she may ask herself are: Is he very thin with only a small amount of subcutaneous tissue to cushion bony prominences? Or is he overweight with much adipose tissue which can help contribute to the problem of pressure over bony prominences? The nurse will want to know what the patient's diet habits have been and to what extent they may be influenced by the present illness. The nurse must know whether the patient is consuming the food which is served to him or if the patient is not eating, she must ascertain the reason and use this information in seeking a solution to the problem.

Another preventive measure is provision for frequent changes of position with protection of susceptible areas from undue pressure. The use of pillows to support the patient in positions which he is unable to maintain will insure the relief of pressure on bony prominences. To be sure that the bed is kept free of irritating agents such as wrinkles or any hard objects, the nurse must include the elimination of such factors as a part of her care when she changes the position of her patients. Prolonged pressure on a specific area interferes with the circulation to that area, resulting in blanching. When the pressure is removed and circulation is restored, the part may become reddened. When the nurse detects changes in the appearance of the skin where pressure has been exerted, she can help to restore the circulation by gentle massage of the area and the use of some lubricating body lotion. Particular attention should be given to the protection of reddened areas from further irritation.

If skin breakdown and ulcer formation occur, the need for constant care and observation is increased. In the presence of skin breakdown and ulcer formation, cleanliness is of utmost importance to promote healing. The nurse will be directed to cleanse the area, sometimes according to a prescribed procedure which calls for use of special cleansing agents. Care must be taken to avoid the use of materials which may predispose further insult to the area. As this cleansing is done, the nurse must observe for changes in the size, shape, and general appearance of the ulcer. This information is essential for evaluation of the method of treatment being employed.

SPECIAL DIAGNOSTIC STUDIES

Patients having special diagnostic studies, such as x-rays, electrocardiogram, electroencephalogram, and metabolic studies, comprise a group of patients whose needs are overlooked frequently. Possible reasons for this negligence may be the fact that, as yet, no diagnosis has been specified. They are usually ambulatory and are able to meet most of their own physical needs, and in fact, some of them may be people who have just come to the hospital specifically for the studies. None of these reasons, however, eliminates the need for certain considerations and care by the nursing and/or technical personnel who happen to come in contact with the patient.

Using the knowledge that she has about the various procedures and the problems which necessitate them, the nurse must observe these patients and offer assistance whenever it is needed. She should make every effort to help the patient to be as comfortable as possible in his particular situation. For example, patients should not be left sitting in drafty hallways with improper clothing. Neither should patients just be left sitting without any introduction to anyone who will be responsible for their care. Patients have said that the most unpleasant part of a diagnostic study was the lack of direction and consideration shown to them as individuals. Sometimes, these patients tend to suspect the worst that can happen. Therefore, they should be kept informed of what is being done so that they will be less worried about the outcomes. Another complaint heard from patients who are having studies is the lack of respect shown for their modesty. Regardless of the sex of the patient, the nurse should see to it that appropriate covering is available for the patient at all times.

Prerequisite to any diagnostic procedure is the need for a careful explanation of what is to happen to the patient and just what he is expected to do. No longer do people see medical and nursing personnel as the only ones who should know what is happening to the patient. Patients read lay literature; through this and through conversations with others, they glean many bits of information, or misinformation, with the result that they come into the hospital with preconceived ideas which may or may not be helpful. If the right to know what is happening is respected and information is provided to the patient, his ability to cooperate will be increased.

Nurses must use good judgment in providing information to patients. It is only reasonable to expect that some patients will have more understanding of themselves and of their illness than others will, and these will be the ones who will need more detailed information. Patients who are unable to understand specific information should not be confused with information which might cause them to be more fearful than before. Caution should always be exerted to insure communication between the nursing and the medical staffs so that each is aware of information given to the patient.

To consider a specific situation, when a patient is to be studied for gastrointestinal problems, the usual preparation consists of withholding food, medications, and water for a specified period prior to the examination. If he has been receiving medication to relieve gastric distress, the chances of his experiencing some discomfort during the fasting period will be increased. If the patient is told exactly how long the procedure will take and how long he must be without medication, he will be able to relax to a greater extent than if he is left to worry and wonder without receiving any instructions. Some patients will be unable to wait the required time for medication, and permission to give medication must be obtained.

Patients who have received harsh laxatives in preparation for studies of the lower intestinal tract may react so severely to the medication that diarrhea will develop. If this occurs, the patient should be observed for undue weakness and should be assisted to the bathroom to protect him from injury. This is a common problem when studies of the lower gastrointestinal tract are being conducted.

When patients are scheduled for any of the electrical studies, such as the electrocardiogram or electroencephalogram, they will be taken to a special unit which has been equipped to do these studies, if their condition permits. Again, patients who are scheduled for electroencephalogram will have medications withheld for twenty-four hours prior to the study. These patients must be observed for any signs of muscle twitching, loss of consciousness, or seizures. If severe symptoms develop, it might be necessary to administer some medication. While medications are not withheld prior to electrocardiograms, the technician and the physician who will interpret the tracing need to know what medications the patient is receiving. It is not uncommon for patients who are having any of the electrical studies to have some fears about the use of the electricity. Careful explanations will help the patient to relax and will help to dispel his fears of electrical shock.

RESPONSIBILITIES FOR LABORATORY STUDIES

There is, as yet, some disagreement over the exact amount of knowledge of basic science required for a nurse to perform her functions. If she is to understand the significance of the various diagnostic studies which are performed in the hospital laboratory, a background knowledge of physiology and body chemistry is essential. It is not necessary to know the procedure for performing the laboratory studies since there are skilled technicians to do them. But the nurse should have some knowledge of the so-called "normal" values of the most commonly ordered studies and the significance of deviations.

Perhaps the most frequently ordered diagnostic studies are those which are ordered almost routinely upon admission of the patient. They are the erythrocyte and leukocyte counts, the hemoglobin and/or hematocrit, urinalysis, and fasting blood sugar. The normal range for the erythrocyte count is from four to five and one-half million cells per cubic milliliter. The leukocyte count ranges from five to six thousand per cubic milliliter.

The hemoglobin and hematocrit levels both indicate the capacity of the red blood cells to transport oxygen. For this reason, the nurse should recognize deviations from the normal ranges of twelve to fourteen grams per hundred milliliters of blood for the hemoglobin level and from thirty-eight to forty-four cubic milliliters of packed cells per hundred milliliters of whole blood for hematocrit. If a nurse notices that her patient seems very tired after minimal activity, she may discover, upon checking his laboratory reports, that he has a low hemoglobin value. This could reduce the amount of energy that his body is able to create due to his decreased ability to transport the oxygen essential for the metabolic process to produce energy.

Even as the nurse collects the specimen for a urinalysis, she can make certain observations of the characteristics of the urine. Knowing that urine is normally clear and straw-colored, variations in either of these characteristics should be noted. Any evidence of cloudiness may be suggestive of some urinary tract infection. The presence of blood in the urine is abnormal and should be brought to the attention of the physician. The nurse should be able to differentiate between urine that is concentrated and urine which contains waste products from the liver, normally excreted through the intestinal tract. The presence of this waste material in the urine causes it to be a very deep amber which is darker than urine that is concentrated.

When a patient has a fasting blood sugar determination, the nurse will be able to observe and care for that patient more intelligently if she is able to compare what is found with the value to be expected in a healthy state. Certain variations suggest the possibility of specific problems in the care of the patient. If the patient has a report of a fasting blood sugar which is far above the normal range, the nurse would know that steps should be taken to counteract hyperglycemia, and she would be able to contact the physician for direction before serious consequences occur.

Another example of patients whose problem might be detected much faster if the nurse were able to recognize signs of deviations are the patients with electrolyte disturbances, especially calcium and potassium. The informed nurse will know that the symptoms of edema, diuresis, alterations of respiratory cycle, and muscle twitching could indicate electrolyte imbalance, and early attention to this matter can prevent more serious problems.[3]

Another study which is ordered frequently is the blood urea and nitrogen level. This test is particularly important in the presence of any impaired function of the kidney and in patients who have suffered severe injuries with extensive tissue damage. Markedly elevated blood levels of these waste products of metabolism can cause disturbance in the orientation of the patient and can eventually lead to such severe cerebral disturbance that the patient is rendered unconscious. The nurse should be familiar with the normal range of this level which is generally considered to be eight to eighteen milligrams of the urea and nitrogen in each one hundred cubic centimeters of blood.

---

[3]Matheney and others, *op. cit.*, page 290.

When the nurse has developed this kind of knowledge, she will realize the importance of reading laboratory reports when they are returned. It is not enough for her to perform only the clerical function of filing the report in the proper place among the many pages of the patient's record. She must read the result of the test so that she will be alerted to the appropriate action. It is, of course, unlikely and unnecessary for the nurse to remember all of the numerical values for the many diagnostic tests that can be performed, but she should become familiar enough with those that are done most often to recognize deviations. With experience and study, the nurse will learn the characteristics of various disorders sufficiently so that a diagnosis, even though tentative, will alert her to signals for which she should observe the patient.

ASSISTING WITH REMOVAL OF FLUID FROM BODY CAVITIES

In the care and treatment of some patients, it becomes necessary to remove fluid or tissue specimens from body parts or cavities for diagnostic purposes or for the relief of pressure. In order to reach into the area in question, special needles or trochars are used. Care must be taken to protect the patient from introduction of pathogenic organisms when any of these procedures are performed. The nurse should be sure that the equipment is sterile and that proper protection is afforded the wound. In addition to preparing the equipment and the patient for the procedures, there are some observations which are relative to the specific procedures.

When fluid is removed from the pleural space, the procedure is called a thoracentesis. When the patient sees the equipment for this procedure, he may become quite alarmed and fearful that he will be harmed by the instruments. He should be told that a local anesthetic will be used and that the procedure will not produce lasting injury or discomfort. It is not a good idea to tell a patient that a procedure "will not hurt at all" or "that he will not feel a thing." Even when local anesthetics are used, there may be an awareness of mild discomfort or pressure over the affected area. If a patient is fearful of injury, even the slightest pressure or discomfort may seem like pain to him. If the patient knows that he can expect these sensations, he will be more able to relax when they do occur. If they do not occur, he will be pleased to know that there was less discomfort than he had anticipated.

As the nurse works with the patient, she can ascertain by her observations whether he is frightened. Adults usually do not like to admit fear, and they may attempt to conceal it by reinforcing the idea that they are not afraid. Through careful and tactful instruction and redirection of attention, the nurse will be able to relieve some of the fear that may be present. When a patient is frightened at the outset of a procedure, he is more likely to become tense, thus adding to the discomfort caused by the procedure.

In addition to observing for undue anxiety about the procedure, there are some physical signs for which the nurse should observe the patient. It is important to check the pulse rate before the procedure to establish a norm for this patient so that variations during the procedure can be detected. The pulse rate can be expected to increase in the presence of fear or excitement. Probably one of the best illustrations of changes in the pulse rate due to excitement can be seen in the records of the astronauts as they performed their daring and exciting responsibilities. While it is true that there are other factors involved which produce changes in their heart rates, it is believed that excitement is responsible for some of the increase.

Respirations should be observed, also, for rate and character. Some patients exhibit their anxiety through changes in the respiratory pattern. Long, sighing respirations with a long expiratory phase may be associated with excitement or anxiety and, if they persist, may cause the patient to become faint. This type of breathing produces hyperventilation with excessive excretion of carbon dioxide. Fainting occurs then because sufficient carbon dioxide for respiratory stmulation is not retained and the body reacts in order to restore its equilibrium.

Patients who are undergoing a thoracentesis, removal of fluid from the pleural space, should be instructed to cease breathing momentarily as the needle is being inserted. They should be instructed to refrain from coughing during the insertion of the needle to prevent injury to the visceral pleura. Penetration of the visceral pleura conceivably can cause the complication of pneumothorax as the opening could permit air from the lung to escape into the pleural space after the thoracentesis is completed. When the external opening caused by the introduction of the needle is sealed off, this air would have no outlet and pressure would increase in the pleural space until it eventually could cause collapse of the lung. Such a collection of air within the pleural space changes the pressure present therein and interferes with respiration. Maintenance of a negative pressure in the pleural space is essential for inspiration to occur.

Observation of the patient's face and hands during a thoracentesis will provide evidence of circulatory changes. Changes most likely to occur would be either flushing or pallor. The patient may perspire as a result of his anxiety. In addition to observing the extent of perspiration, the nurse can help the patient to relax by simply offering him a cloth to wipe his brow or by wiping his forehead for him if he is unable to do this for himself. Anticipation of needs such as this communicates to the patient that he is being carefully protected and, thus, will help him to relax as he feels more secure.

Following the procedure of thoracentesis, the patient should be assisted into a comfortable position and instructed to rest quietly for an hour or so. During this time, he should be observed for any difficulty with respiration. Unless the patient appears to be having difficulty, the pulse usually is not checked.

The only dressing required for the wound caused by the insertion of the needle will be a small dressing such as a band-aid. Sometimes, no covering is used. The nurse should check the area for any evidence of bleeding. While it is unlikely that bleeding will occur, it is a possibility, and early detection will prevent serious problems.

Observation of fluid obtained from thoracentesis includes measurement of the amount and noting of its color and consistency. Unless specifically directed, the nurse should retain the entire specimen and send it with the proper requests to the laboratory for analysis.

Removal of fluid from the abdominal cavity is called paracentesis. This procedure is done usually for the purpose of relieving pressure on the viscera and/or abdominal wall. In some medical disorders, the abdominal circulation becomes inadequate and fluid accumulates in the peritoneal cavity. This is a particular problem for patients with abdominal malignancies and those with cirrhosis of the liver. The nurse should pay particular attention to the size and hardness of the abdomen as she is caring for any patients with these diagnoses. If and when the physician elects to perform a paracentesis, the nurse will need to instruct the patient as to his role during the procedure. Again, the nurse should observe the patient for any sign of undue fatigue or anxiety such as excessive perspiration, pallor, trembling fingers or shaky hands, and changes in respirations. Although the patient may indicate that he prefers to watch the procedure, he may tolerate it better if his attention is directed elsewhere until the procedure has been completed.

Because of the amount of fluid removed through this treatment, the procedure may require considerably more time than some others. Sometimes, as much as four or five liters of fluid are removed. Because of the quantity, the nurse will want to have a large receptacle readily available.

The patient will need to be in a sitting position for this procedure. If he is able, the nurse can assist the patient into a chair so that he will have adequate foot and back support or she can help him to sit on the side of the bed and place pillows behind him for support. It is important that the patient is well supported because he will grow tired before the procedure is completed.

Characteristics of the fluid to be observed and recorded will be the color, consistency, and quantity. Disposition should be at the direction of the physician. Again, the total quantity should be reserved until the physician decides what portion he wishes to have sent to the laboratory or reserved for some other reason. The color of fluid obtained from the abdominal cavity should be pale yellow or straw colored. The fluid should appear clear and somewhat more viscous than water.

Because of the size of the trochar used for this procedure, sometimes the physician will use one or two sutures to insure proper closure of the wound. A small dressing should then be applied to protect the area from gross contamination. The nurse should check for any evidence of bleeding for the next hour or two.

Patients who are to have a spinal tap or lumbar puncture may or may not be apprehensive. If the patient knows this procedure requires the introduction of a needle into the spinal canal, he may be quite fearful that the spinal cord will be injured or that he will experience severe pain as a result of the procedure. Instructions about what is expected of the patient, the position he will assume, and the importance of his remaining still throughout the procedure should help to allay some of the fears. Care should be taken to assist the patient into a comfortable position before the procedure is initiated.

The purpose of the spinal tap or lumbar puncture may be to obtain fluid for special examination or to determine the pressure existing in the spinal canal. Pressure is especially important in patients with problems involving the brain such as tumors, injuries, or obstruction of the path of the spinal fluid. Because of the rigidity of its structure, there is no means of relieving this pressure, and continued increase can produce serious injury to the brain tissue. Characteristics of the fluid are especially important if there is suspicion of bleeding anywhere within the cranium or if infection is suspected. Before sending the specimen to the laboratory, the nurse must make a note of her observations. A band-aid or other small bandage will be sufficient to cover the wound. The bandage can be removed after a few hours when the wound has had sufficient time to seal itself and the nurse has ascertained that no bleeding is present. Protection of the wound from contamination by pathogenic organisms is the most important reason for the bandage.

When such procedures as the bone marrow biopsy and pericardial tap are ordered, the nurse's main concern will be the supportive care and observation of the patient. As with the previously discussed procedures, care should be taken to protect the patient from contamination of the wound and to maintain as much comfort as possible. For bone marrow biopsy, a small container with a preservative fluid will be required to receive the specimen. For pericardial tap, the amount of fluid obtained will be small but the exact amount should be determined. Sterile equipment will be needed for both of these procedures. Patient instructions will be similar to those given for any other intrusive procedure. After-care will consist of disposition of the specimen and observation of the patient for any untoward reaction.

Two other procedures which deserve consideration here are the liver and kidney biopsy. As their names imply, both are done for diagnostic purposes. These procedures are discussed together because of the similarity of the complications that can arise and the observations to be made. Because of the vascularity of both of these organs, the greatest danger is of bleeding following the procedure. Since there is such a danger of trauma to the vessels of these organs and to the organs themselves, the patient will be required to stay in bed for several hours after completion of the procedure. The exact length of time will vary from one hospital to another.

During the period of bedrest, the nurse will be expected to observe the blood pressure, pulse, and respirations at intervals to be ordered by the physician. These readings should be recorded on a graph so that, from a glance, the physician can tell exactly what the pattern is. If bleeding should occur following either of these procedures, the blood pressure and pulse would be the most reliable indicators. In the event of bleeding, surgical intervention may be required to correct the problem. Other indications of internal hemorrhage are thirst, apprehension, and change in skin color to pallor or to cyanosis which results from inadequate peripheral circulation.

Although joint aspirations do not fall into the same category as penetrations of the body cavities, the joints do represent closed areas which are susceptible to infection if contaminated. Some diseases cause acute inflammation of the joints and may produce fluid accumulation within the joint capsule. The purpose for joint aspiration may be to relieve the pressure caused by the accumulation of fluid or to obtain a specimen for laboratory examination and diagnosis. The same precautions of sterile technique during and after the procedure should be observed. Also, the area should be observed for any bleeding following the procedure. Disposition of the specimen should be carried out in accordance with the direction of the physician.

ADMINISTERING MEDICATIONS

Preparation and administration of medications does not complete the nursing responsibilities related to drug therapy. From the earliest experience with medications, the nurse is taught the importance of administering drugs accurately and waiting to see that the patient actually takes his medication. Some hospitals are introducing new systems in which patients who are able are permitted to keep their medications at their bedsides and take them as directed. Even in situations such as this, the nurse has a responsibility beyond providing the necessary medications and equipment for the actual administration. That responsibility is the observation of the patient for the effects of the drug.

In order to determine the effectiveness of a drug, the nurse must know exactly what medication the patient has had. The following patient situation is presented as an example of careless and inadequate nursing care.

> Upon entering Mrs. G's room, the nurse observed that Mrs. G was looking for a wastebasket in which to deposit a small white cup. As the nurse offered assistance, Mrs. G commented that this paper cup had contained some medication and that she had just taken it. She had found the cup sitting on her bedside stand when she awakened from an afternoon nap and, assuming that it had been left for her, proceeded to swallow its contents.

While patients should receive credit for their intellect and ability, the fallacy in the above situation is in the lack of communication with the patient about the medication. Patients should not be expected to awaken and swallow whatever may be left at the bedside. It is possible that the patient may swallow something that is not intended for ingestion. Also, provision must be made for evaluation of the effectiveness of the drug.

Whenever a nurse administers medications, she should have some knowledge about the action of the drug, the purpose for which this patient is receiving it, and any untoward effects which might be anticipated. In this day, when most people have received one or more of the recently developed antibiotics, there is a high incidence of sensitivity to these drugs. Dangers associated with these sensitivities require the nurse to know about her patient's history of allergies and any medications received. Allergic reactions are not to be considered lightly. They may be manifested by mild symptoms at first, but subsequent reactions may be characterized by more drastic effects. The use of some type of signaling system for marking the charts of patients with known allergies is essential and should be heeded rigidly.

Observations pertaining to medication begin with the actual preparation of the medication. As the nurse's knowledge of drugs grows, she will develop some knowledge of the general characteristics of the most frequently administered drugs. It must be remembered, however, that different manufacturers may prepare the same drug with different external characteristics, so one must read labels carefully when preparing medications for administration. When the medication contained in a bottle appears different from the kind that has been in the bottle before, the nurse should consult the pharmacist before administering it. She may learn that the difference is only in its appearance because it comes from a different manufacturer.

Observable reactions of drugs depend upon the type of drug and the purpose for which it is given. If a patient receives an antipyretic, the nurse must know that its purpose is to reduce the body temperature, and therefore, she must check the temperature after a half or three-quarters of an hour has passed in order to determine the effectiveness of the drug. When patients have pain which requires the administration of analgesics, the nurse should return to see if the pain has been relieved.

The action of antibiotics is not observed as rapidly as the action of some other drugs, but the appearance of urticaria, edema, or rash following administration of antibiotics should be recognized as signs of a possible allergic reaction. Any subsequent doses of the medication should be withheld until the physician has had an opportunity to examine the reaction. Some patients are highly sensitive to antibiotics, and the reaction can occur rapidly causing the patient to suffer anaphylactic shock.

When medications are given to induce sleep, it is important to observe the patient to evaluate the effectiveness of the drug. In some cases, an order will be provided for additional doses if the first one is inadequate. When the nurse returns to evaluate the effectiveness of sedatives, she must exercise caution to avoid disturbing the patient, but she must not assume that everyone who is lying quietly is sleeping.

When a rapid effect is desired from a medication, the drug may be given by a parenteral route. Drugs given intravenously, intramuscularly, or subcutaneously produce a more rapid effect than drugs that are ingested orally.[4] The reason for this is that the drug reaches the circulatory system more quickly and consequently is transported to its site of action more rapidly. The amount of time required for the action of these drugs is reduced, and the effectiveness can be evaluated earlier.

---

[4]Martha Pitel and Mary Wemmett, "The Intramuscular Injection," *American Journal of Nursing*, Vol. 64, No. 4, 1964, page 104.

Some drugs require much more constant observation of patients because of their potency. An example of this is levophed bitartrate* which is given intravenously for the purpose of increasing the blood pressure. The patient will receive the drug by continuous drip, the rate of which will be regulated according to the blood level. Frequent measurement of the blood pressure will be necessary because of the marked fluctuations which can be produced by this drug. Levophed bitartrate also is a dangerous drug in its action upon body tissue, and for this reason, the site at which the needle enters the vein must be observed closely for the development of infiltration of this substance into the surrounding tissue. When it is discovered early, an antidote can be injected which decreases the severity of its action upon the subcutaneous tissues. Skin grafts have been necessitated by the wounds produced by the effects of levophed bitartrate escaping into the tissue surrounding the vein which was punctured.

Administration of some medications is regulated by the results of specific laboratory tests. When such is the case, as with the anticoagulants, the nurse must see to it that the report of the study is obtained from the laboratory. Another example would be the patient who has diabetes and whose dosage of insulin is being regulated. The amount of insulin that he will receive daily will vary according to his body needs, as demonstrated through blood glucose levels and urine reductions. The order for insulin will be written so that the dose for a specific time will be determined by the presence of sugar and/or acetone in the urine. Accurate observation and interpretation of urine reductions then is essential.

When self-medication is permitted as with nitroglycerine for patients who suffer attacks of angina, the nurse must obtain information from the patient about the attacks as well as furnishing an adequate supply of the medication. For any patient receiving medications, a record is essential to show the medications administered, the time and route of administration, and any results observed. Such a record may serve as a clue in the detection of sensitivity reactions. The possibility of untoward reaction to any medication such as nausea, vomiting, rash, or other unexpected results must be remembered. If such side effects occur, the physician should know so that he can alter his therapy accordingly.

Medications differ in their actions and in the time required to produce their effects. Regardless of the medication being given, the nurse must know the purpose for which it is being given, the approximate

---

*Trade name for levarterenol bitartrate.

length of time required for its action, and the symptoms of any adverse reaction. With new drugs being developed every day, it is impossible for a nurse to know everything about all of them, but no nurse should be willing to give a medication without first learning these basic facts regarding it.

ASSISTING WITH INTRAVENOUS THERAPY

Use of intravenous therapy has contributed greatly to the successful treatment of patients whose lives may have been lost otherwise. It is possible to administer life saving medications, fluids, electrolytes, and nutrients through this route when the patient is unable to ingest anything through the alimentary route. While this therapy can produce dramatic effects, it is not free of hazards. When adverse reactions occur, they occur so rapidly that immediate action is necessary. For this reason, someone must be constantly on guard for signals of their development. Since nursing personnel are in the most constant attendance, this becomes a prime nursing responsibility. The nurse must become so familiar with this therapy and the signals which call for attention that her observation becomes an almost automatic behavior. From the time the equipment is assembled until the therapy is completed, there must be thoughtful surveillance.

Although the actual venipuncture was left to the physician for many years, more and more nurses are being taught to administer this therapy except when blood or plasma is to be administered.[5] For the purpose of clarity, blood transfusions will be discussed separately. When intravenous therapy is ordered, the nurse's first responsibility will be to assemble all of the equipment needed to carry out this procedure. If medications are to be added to the sterile solutions, the nurse must be sure that they are added in such a way that contamination of the fluid does not occur. The addition of medications must be carried out in accordance with hospital policy. Some hospitals delegate only to specific individuals the privilege, or responsibility, of adding sterile medications to solutions which are to be administered intravenously. Such limitations are imposed for the protection of the patient.

As the nurse assembles the equipment, she must examine the containers of the sterile fluids to be administered to be sure that the seals are intact. Any cloudiness of solution would suggest contamination and, therefore, it should not be used. She must exercise due caution to avoid contamination as she connects the tubing to the fluid container

---

[5]*Intravenous Therapy Manual* (Harrisburg, Pennsylvania: The Pennsylvania Nurses Association, 1960), page 2.

and prepares the needle which is to be inserted into the patient's vein. Observations of any break in technique should be called to the attention of the person performing this treatment, if the nurse is assisting.

Care must be taken to remove all air from the tubing to prevent the introduction of air into the patient's vein. If air is injected into the vein, it becomes an embolus which could incur harmful effects to the patient. Once the needle has been inserted and the flow of fluid has been established, the nurse is responsible for maintaining a constant watch over the patient. Whenever a nurse sees a patient receiving intravenous therapy, regardless of whether he is assigned to her for care, she should respond automatically. Her response should be to notice whether the fluid is dripping continuously into the drip chamber and at what rate it is dripping. It requires less than a minute to determine the rate of flow.

When the nurse observes that the fluid is dripping either too slowly or too rapidly, she must investigate more closely to ascertain the problem and to correct it. When fluids are given too rapidly, patients who have impaired circulation can develop pulmonary edema. If the fluid is dripping too slowly, the patient may be required to have the treatment prolonged unnecessarily. Such mechanical factors as a kink in the tubing or disturbance of the needle which has caused it either to penetrate the opposite wall of the vein or to be withdrawn from the site of injection can interfere with the flow of fluid. If the needle has become dislodged, the fluid will flow into the tissues and produce a cold, indurated area surrounding the site at which the needle enters the skin. This condition is known as infiltration. The area surrounding the site of injection should be examined for any leakage of fluid which can be detected by the presence of wet bandages, clothing, or linens near the area. If infiltration does occur, the nurse should follow the recommended procedure according to hospital policy. If the nurse is authorized to administer intravenous therapy, she could proceed to remove the needle and, after replacing it with a sterile needle, restart the fluid therapy in another vein. If the nurse is not authorized to do this, she should simply discontinue the fluid therapy either by closing the clamp to interrupt the flow of fluid or by removing the needle and then notifying the person who is authorized to restart the therapy.

Another observation that the nurse should make automatically pertains to amount of fluid left in the bottles. If only a small amount remains, she should check the physician's order to determine whether the therapy is almost completed or if more fluid is to be added. Additional bottles should be hung early enough to prevent the entrance of air into the tubing as the last of the fluid drains from the bottle.

The nurse should observe the patient for any signs of untoward reactions to medications which have been added to the fluid. Although the incidence of reactions may not be very high, they are always serious and are potentially harmful to the patient. Such reactions might be expected to occur within a short time following institution of the therapy because of the introduction of the allergen directly into the vein. Rapid steps must be taken to counteract such reactions, so time is vitally important.

ASSISTING WITH BLOOD TRANSFUSIONS

In addition to the precautions to be taken in assembling the equipment for routine intravenous therapy, there are others which pertain specifically to the administration of blood or plasma. The laboratory technician will obtain a specimen of the patient's blood for typing and crossmatching. When blood is brought to the unit for administration to a patient, it will have been labelled clearly for a specific patient. The nurse must check the name and blood type before delivering the blood to the physician who is to start the transfusion. Hospital policy may require the physician to check the blood for proper identification and to initiate the flow of the blood. Once the transfusion has been started, the nurse must observe for the same factors as for any intravenous therapy with the additional observation for symptoms of incompatibility.

With more complete knowledge about the nature of blood, tests have been developed which decrease markedly the possibility of giving incompatible blood to patients. However, in spite of the more exact matching, reactions do occur. Some symptoms of reactions are chills, complaints of not feeling well, and the appearance of urticaria. When a patient expresses any of these complaints, he should be given immediate attention. The nurse should tighten the clamp on the tubing to interrupt the flow of blood into the patient's vein and contact the physician who will determine the exact nature of the problem. This applies also for problems that occur with the administration of plasma, packed cells, or plasma expanders.

Some hospitals have a standing policy that any remaining blood be returned to the laboratory for further examination and that a urine specimen be obtained the following morning. The urine is examined for the presence of blood which may result from the damaging effects of the sensitivity reaction. Kidney damage can occur with severe reaction to blood transfusion. Transfusion reactions are recorded on the patient's chart, and a record is kept by the laboratory. When no untoward reaction occurs, the nurse must record her observations of the patient's ability to tolerate this treatment.

ADMINISTERING ENEMAS

When a physician orders an enema to be administered to a patient, there are certain observations which the nurse should make. As she works, she should observe the ability of the patient to tolerate the procedure. Sometimes, patients become weak, nauseated, or extremely uncomfortable and are unable to endure the entire procedure. If such is the case, the nurse should cease the procedure and consult the physician for the next move.

When the patient expels the enema, the nurse should observe the results for any unusual characteristics of the amount, consistency, color, and presence of mucus, blood, or any other foreign material. A comment describing the results should be entered in the nursing notes. The presence of hemorrhoids should be checked later to detect any untoward effects that may have occurred.

CATHETERIZATION

In the presence of some urinary tract problems and whenever a patient is unable to void of his own volition, catheterization may be indicated to remove the contents of the bladder. When catherterization is ordered, it must be carried out as a sterile procedure due to the fact that the inside of the bladder is a sterile field. In fact, catheterization is avoided whenever possible to guard against the introduction of infection into the bladder.

When urine is removed from the bladder by means of a catheter, the amount and characteristics should be noted. The presence of any blood, pus, mucus, or other unusual material should be noted and brought to the attention of the physician. Caution is advised when the bladder is distended, and it is recommended that no more than 800 to 1000 c.c. of urine be removed initially. If more urine is removed, the sudden collapse of the bladder wall may cause loss of bladder tone with the further result that the patient will continue having difficulty emptying the bladder. For obvious reasons, when male patients must be catheterized, either the physician, male nurse, or technician will perform the task.

Whenever it is necessary to leave the catheter in place, personnel working with the patient must be taught that the tubing leading to the drainage bottle must be maintained as a closed, sterile system. It is, therefore, important that the tubing be protected from undue stress as well as from contamination when the drainage bottle must be emptied.

APPLICATION OF HEAT

The nurse may be called upon to apply heat to a part of the body for relief of pain or in the treatment of inflammation. When this treatment is ordered, the physician will order the method of application whether it be hot water bottle, electric heating pad, application of warm compresses, or some other method. Regardless of the method, the nurse must observe the area to be treated, its response to the treatment, and the condition of the equipment to be used.

Remembering that water is a better conductor of heat than air, the recommended method must be followed meticulously. If one of the dry methods is to be used, caution must be taken to protect the skin surface from any moisture. In order to prevent burns, a layer of protective material should be used between either the heating pad or hot water bottle and the skin. Care must be taken to apply heat at the recommended temperature and only for the recommended length of time. While it is not the purpose here to discuss the effects of heat, the fact that patients can be burned by overexposure does exist. Although redness will occur as vasodilation is produced, the natural skin color will return after the source of heat has been removed. The area should be examined later for any evidence of a burn.

The same precautions and observations are necessary when moist heat is applied. The main difference between application of dry and moist heat is that with moist heat the part being treated comes in direct contact with the heat. The additional consideration of sterility may be a factor if an open lesion is being treated. Any drainage from a wound being treated with heat should be handled carefully to prevent spread of infection to the nurse or to other patients.

APPLICATION OF COLD

Application of cold to a part is usually done for the purpose of controlling bleeding or swelling or relieving pain. Prolonged application of cold to an area can produce injury, so strict adherence to directions is essential. Whenever cold is being applied to an area, the part receiving the treatment should be observed carefully beforehand to detect the presence of any bleeding, drainage, or other evidence of difficulty. A layer of dry, protective material should be placed between the cooling agent and the skin.

When the treatment has been completed, observation should continue to determine the effectiveness of the treatment. If cold has been applied to relieve pain, the nurse must learn from the patient whether the treatment has been effective. All of these observations should be clearly and concisely recorded.

SUPERVISION OF MECHANICAL EQUIPMENT AND PATIENT SAFETY

As more complex equipment is being employed in the care of the sick, a patient's room sometimes takes on the appearance of a physics or electrical engineering laboratory. Many nursing curricula now require students to have an introduction to the basic laws of physics to enable them to understand more clearly the operation of some of the more commonly used machines. Even so, nurses cannot begin to understand all of the details of these machines. Their role is to learn the location and meaning of the indicators which provide information as to the proper functioning of the machine.

For example, if a patient has a drainage tube inserted into the chest following surgery, the nurse must know that one means of determining that the system is working properly is the increase in the amount of drainage in the bottle. The application of an adhesive strip at premeasured intervals will serve as a guide to the rate of flow of drainage. The chest drainage bottles represent a system which deserves another type of consideration, too. If the nurse knows what gravity is, she can learn its importance in the creation of a gentle suction to help remove drainage from the chest cavity. Knowledge of this principle will enable her to see to it that no one raises the bottles from the floor level.

When any electrical machinery is being used in the care of patients, the nurse must understand that the safety of the patient depends upon proper functioning of the machinery. Wires should always be protected and out of the path of anyone who comes near the patient to avoid hazards to the patient and to those who are responsible for his care. In the interest of patient safety, any defective equipment should be reported immediately and used again only after necessary repairs have been made.

When oxygen equipment is being used, the room should be marked with the caution to refrain from smoking in the area. Additional protection should be afforded the patient by removing any matches from his room. This is not intended to underestimate the intelligence of a patient, but it must be remembered that, when under stress, people react differently than under normal circumstances. If a person is usually a heavy smoker, it is quite possible that he could reach for a cigarette and attempt to light it before he thinks about the presence of oxygen equipment. It is a fact that oxygen does not burn itself, but it does support combustion sufficiently to cause a sudden flash of fire which could injure the patient seriously, if not fatally.

Another vital piece of equipment is the fire extinguisher. Nurses should discipline themselves to become familiar with the location of the fire extinguishers so that time would not be wasted in the event of fire. The nurse must know the location of all emergency equipment on her unit so that she can act quickly in the event of any emergency.

A part of the orientation program to most hospitals is the evacuation system. Although much of the enthusiasm for developing evacuation plans has been generated by the fears of nuclear disasters, it should be emphasized that such plans can prove beneficial in the face of any number of natural disasters such as floods or storms which may cause damages leading to fire. Evacuation plans are not to be regarded lightly, and spare time could be spent wisely reading the plans posted in conspicuous places throughout the hospital.

SUMMARY

The importance of the need to use purposefully all of the time spent with patients cannot be overemphasized. The performance of the nursing activities required in the care of the sick provide the nurse with many opportunities to observe the patient. This chapter has been concerned with observations to be made in specific situations.

BIBLIOGRAPHY

ADRIANI, JOHN, "Venipuncture," *American Journal of Nursing*, Vol. 62, No. 1, 1962, p. 66-70.

BERMOSK, LORETTA SUE, and MORDAN, MARY JANE, *Interviewing in Nursing*. New York: The Macmillan Company, 1964.

BERTHIAUNE, AILEEN B., "Observing Is More Than Watching," *Nursing Outlook*, Vol. 5, No. 5, 1957, p. 290-293.

CROUCH, MADGE L., and GIBSON, SAM T., "Blood Therapy," *American Journal of Nursing*, Vol. 62, No. 3, 1962, p. 71-76.

FRENCH, RUTH M., *Nurse's Guide to Diagnostic Procedures*. New York: Blakiston Division, McGraw-Hill Book Company, 1962.

FUERST, ELINOR V., and WOLFF, LUVERNE, *Fundamentals of Nursing*. Philadelphia: J. B. Lippincott Company, 1964.

HARMER, BERTHA, and HENDERSON, VIRGINIA, *Textbook of the Principles and Practice of Nursing*, 5th ed. New York: The Macmillan Company, 1958.

Intravenous Therapy Manual. Harrisburg, Pennsylvania: The Pennsylvania Nurses Association, 1960.

KLASE, LINDA, and WHALEN, ROBERT, "What Patients Undergoing Cardiac Catheterization Feared," *American Journal of Nursing*, Vol. 62, No. 10, 1962, p. 112-114.

MATHENEY, RUTH V., and others, *Fundamentals of Patient-Centered Nursing.* St. Louis: The C. V. Mosby Company, 1964.

ORLANDO, IDA JEAN, *The Dynamic Nurse-Patient Relationship.* New York: G. P. Putnam's Sons, 1961.

PITEL, MARTHA, and WEMMETT, MARY, "The Intramuscular Injection," *American Journal of Nursing*, Vol. 64, No. 4, 1964, p. 104-109.

SHANCK, ANN H., "The Nurse in An I.V. Therapy Program," *American Journal of Nursing*, Vol. 57, No. 10, 1957, p. 1012-1013.

STILWELL, ELIZABETH HONES, "Pressure Sores," *American Journal of Nursing*, Vol. 64, No. 11, 1964, p. 109-110.

TAYLOR, JOHN C., "Decubitus Ulcers," *Nursing Science*, Vol. 2, No. 4, 1964, p. 293-300.

Chapter _____ 5

Application of Observation
to Patient Situations

Remembering that the overall purpose of this book is to help the student learn to observe the patients for whom she is caring, it seems appropriate now to consider observations to be made in some specific patient situations. While reading this chapter, there may be patients that will be familiar either through individual experience or the shared experience of classmates. It must be understood that the material in this chapter is intended to be an overview of what the nurse can see in a given situation and is not a detailed consideration of the scientific bases for the disorders represented. This type of detailed information will be included in other courses. For the purposes of this discussion, patients have been chosen to represent a variety of general situations. Some of the discussion is centered around groups of patients whose needs are similar by virtue of their age or experience. Other parts of the discussion are related to more specific problems encountered by patients.

THE AMBULATORY PATIENT

Observation of the ambulatory patient poses a problem that is quite different from observing a person who is bedfast. By the very nature of the demands for assistance, less time usually is spent with the ambulatory patient than with the bedfast patient. This is not to say, however, that the need for observation is any less. The fact that the ambulatory patient is able to take care of many of his personal needs reduces the amount of time the nurse may be working directly with him. The tendency in a busy ward situation is to spend only the time needed for direct physical care with patients. Thus, it becomes possible to overlook or to minimize the needs of the ambulatory patients.

Nurses must learn that ambulatory patients have needs, too. The main difference is that their needs are at a different level than the needs of those who are bedridden and who therefore require considerable assistance with basic physiologic needs. The thought of spending time just listening to a patient is disturbing to many nurses because their entire orientation has been directed toward getting things done. As the patient's condition improves, he begins to think about things beyond his hospital room, to plan for his discharge from the hospital, and to think about his return to his social setting. He will wonder how he will manage if he has acquired new limitations and what it will be like to be back on his feet again.

The ambulatory patient may be a person who has just arrived in the hospital for surgical treatment of a known problem or for diagnostic studies to identify a problem which is as yet unknown. People who are having diagnostic studies often are treated as if they are perfectly healthy, happy people. This may not be the case. It must be remembered that no one enters a hospital for pleasure or recreation.

As he ponders the many questions that may arise, the patient will need to discuss them with someone. Perhaps the nurse will not have the answers, but she should never underestimate the help she can give just by offering a small part of her time to listen. As she listens, the nurse may find that a referral is needed for some type of follow-up care or supervision. Or she may find that the patient needs some further instructions regarding his care. Regardless of the need he feels, his needs do deserve consideration. The hospital holds many mysteries to the outsider, adult or child. Those who work inside the hospital become so familiar with its sight, its sounds, and even its odors that their strangeness fades away. A patient entering the hospital cannot feel this way. He has a very personal interest in whatever happens. He knows that his welfare is at stake, and all of the strangeness of the environment may represent threats to him. The nurse should remember that all she needs to do is to treat the ambulatory patient with the same respect as that shown the bedfast patient.

THE PATIENT IN THE OUTPATIENT CLINIC

The scene in an outpatient clinic is usually one of several long, hard benches which are filled with rows of weary patients seeking initial or follow-up care. Some may be accompanied by a friend or relative who has come to assist them and to protect them from mishap. Others have come alone using the only money they have for carfare to and from the clinic. Some patients will appear to be in no acute distress while others may appear to be suffering great discomfort.

For example, the nurse must be alert to the patient who is having difficulty breathing. Perhaps it is only the result of climbing stairs and will pass with a bit of rest, but conversely, it may mean that the patient is having severe problems which are posing a great danger to his welfare. The nurse in the outpatient clinic must be on guard for the diabetic patient who may have withheld his insulin and breakfast so that a fasting blood specimen could be obtained upon his arrival at clinic. Once the specimen is obtained, the nurse must see to it that the patient receives his insulin and some food. Otherwise, she may have to cope with a more serious problem. Then, there may be patients who are weak just because they have not eaten. The nurse should observe the presence of any bandages or prostheses which may require attention. Regardless of his reason for coming to the clinic, the patient should be observed as he waits his turn to be seen by the physician so that problems can be averted.

Through her interview with the patient, the nurse in the outpatient clinic must obtain key information pertaining to the problems related specifically to his illness. This will enable her to help the patient obtain whatever information he needs from the physician. Many patients still tend to hold the physician in such awe that they cannot feel sufficiently at ease to remember the many questions that may be bothering them.

Opportunities for teaching in an outpatient setting are unlimited. Ingenuity, coupled with awareness of need, will enable the nurse to develop teaching devices which can be studied by the patient as he waits his turn to be treated. Explanations given after the patient has been seen by the physician will be instructive, too. No nurse in an outpatient clinic should become so preoccupied with procedures that she loses sight of the tremendous opportunity to exercise her imagination and creativity to help patients. Observation in the outpatient clinic becomes more than observation of signs and symptoms related to illness. It must include the observation of the need for knowledge.

THE PATIENT IN HIS HOME

The concept of public health nursing encompasses a broad area of nursing practice through official and voluntary agencies. While many of these agencies have been in existence for a long time, recent years have witnessed the development of still another plan for the care of the sick at home. These programs are called home-care programs, and they have been established as an extension of hospital services. Such programs have made it possible for patients to go home earlier and thus reduce the cost of their hospital and medical care. Teams of physicians and nurses visit these people in the home to provide the necessary medical care and health supervision. It thus becomes important for nurses to become skilled in the observation of these patients and their home situations.

What does a nurse look for when she visits a patient in his home? Of primary concern will be the actual condition of the patient. The nurse will need to make observations which are specifically related to his progress toward health. The exact nature of these observations will be determined by the problem which necessitated hospitalization. For example, the observation of a patient who has been diagnosed as having diabetes will include such factors as observing the condition of his feet and legs, observing the patient testing a specimen of his urine for the presence of glucose, observing the patient administering his own insulin, observing the handling and care of the equipment used to administer insulin, reviewing with the patient his dietary habits and needs, and the attitude of the patient regarding his health problem and care. Through evaluation of all of these observations, the nurse can determine the extent to which the patient has been able to make necessary adjustments and identify aspects of care with which the patient continues to need assistance. A knowledge of the patient she is to visit and the record of his hospital care will alert the nurse to the particular observations to be made.

The state of health of other members of the family is also important. While it is recognized that the nurse visiting a patient in his home administers care under the direction and supervision of a physician, she is permitted to refer patients to appropriate sources for medical attention when it is needed. Visiting in the home provides an excellent opportunity for the nurse to discern needs which can be met through the various social and health agencies in the community.

As the nurse observes the total family situation, she should make an assessment of the quality of interpersonal relationships in the home. The limitations or special needs of the patient may cause a temporary inconvenience to other members of the family. If other members are unable or unwilling to adjust to these inconveniences, friction may result. For example, when a patient returns home with the dietary restriction that he is permitted no salt, adjustment may be required by all members of the family. This is especially true if the family has been accustomed to having their food seasoned during cooking. Teaching all members of the family of the importance of this change can facilitate their adjustment and can help to maintain good interpersonal relationships.[1]

Physical facilities are also important in the care of a patient at home. While the standard of living is higher today than at any time in the history of the United States, there are still many people who live in homes with very definite health hazards. As the nurse works in the home, she should look specifically at the condition of any stairs, the toilet facilities, the heating system, and provisions for cooking. Unvented gas heaters cause hundreds of deaths due to carbon monoxide poisoning every winter. Broken or cluttered stairs serve as a menace to all who must use them. Handrails are a must for homes where there are children or elderly people. Bathrooms can be made safer by the addition of handrails to be used when getting into or out of the bathtub. Shower stalls should be protected by a slip-proof covering on the floor. Although it may seem that it should be understood without mention, a properly functioning toilet is also a must. Where substandard housing exists, the absence of adequate toilet facilities is not uncommon.

Potential fire hazards should also be identified, and patients and their families should be encouraged to remove them. The nurse should ascertain from the patient and his family what provisions and plan they have for escape in the event of fire. Although the nurse is not expected to be a housing or fire inspector, she must be alert to the existence of any factors which may threaten the safety of her patients.

THE PATIENT RECEIVING RADIOISOTOPE THERAPY

Use of radioisotopes in medicine is becoming more prevalent, and even more extensive use in the future can be anticipated. It becomes important then to understand something about the principles which safeguard nurse, visitor, and patient when this type of therapy is being administered.

It is important to realize, first, that because these patients are assigned a private room with signs posted warning everyone against entry, the number of people who enter will be reduced. Consequently, the patient soon begins to feel himself imprisoned and even rejected by nursing personnel and other patients. For the protection of everyone

[1]Ruth B. Freeman, *Public Health Nursing Practice*, 2nd ed. (Philadelphia: W. B. Saunders Company, 1957), page 95.

concerned, it is necessary to limit those who enter the room to those who have been instructed in the proper handling of items contaminated by radiation. Such restrictions are necessary so that undue contamination by radioactive substances can be prevented. The nurse must look for ways, then, to help this patient accept his therapy without feeling that he is being treated as if he were in some disgraceful situation which causes everyone to pass him by.

Because of the potential danger of exposure to radioactivity, it becomes necessary to isolate the patient who is receiving radioisotope therapy. The care of the patient who is isolated requires hospital personnel to handle and dispose of such items as linens, dishes, and any other equipment used in the care of the patient in such a way that protection of everyone is insured. Receptacles for contaminated items must be labelled clearly and kept within the patient's room until they can be disposed of properly. Carelessness in the handling of radioactive materials can produce serious effects, some of which may not appear for a long time after the exposure to such materials has occurred.

The radiologist in charge of the therapy can provide valuable assistance in this matter. In addition to periodic checking of the room with a Geiger counter to determine the extent of radioactivity, he will be able to offer guidance of all personnel who will be working with the patient. A list of specific instructions will be left in a conspicuous place such as the bulletin board in the nurses' station. Also, signs bearing the commonly accepted symbol of radioactivity will be placed on the patient's chart as well as on the door to his room. Some hospitals use special linens and laundry bags which are identified by color. Any further question concerning the care of the patient should be referred to the radiologist.

As the nurse works with the patient, she should pay particular attention to his mental state. For example, a group of patients who have been treated effectively with radioactive iodine are patients with hyperthyroidism. These patients, because of their physical problem, are already hyperirritable. The limited contact with other patients and nurses can serve to produce even more restlessness and anxiety.

When accompanying a patient for x-ray studies or therapy, the zealous student must not insist that she remain in the presence of the patient because there is danger of repeated exposure to the x-rays. Repeated exposure to x-rays can produce harmful effects. The technician will be happy to explain what is being done and why, so that learning objectives can be achieved. If the presence of the nurse is required, she should obtain appropriate protective apparel from the technician.

THE PATIENT UNDERGOING SURGERY

The Preoperative Patient

Except for people who require emergency surgery, patients enter the hospital at least one day prior to the date of their surgery so that certain preparations and observations can be made. Many of the observations to be made by the nurse upon admission are the same as for any newly admitted patient. But there are some additional factors which must be kept in mind.

It is the unusual patient who enters the hospital for surgery with no fears about his coming experiences. Although he may present an outward appearance of self-confidence, it is quite likely that, regardless of his problem or knowledge, he will have some apprehension about his surgery and the possible outcomes. He may have fears pertaining to pain, anesthesia, finance, the welfare of his family, the hospital regime, or even death. While it is not a good idea to suggest things for the patient to worry about, the nurse should try to evaluate his attitude as she works with him and should provide opportunities for him to express any fears that he might have. She must listen carefully as she converses with her patient so she can respond to any clues that he may offer. It is important to remember that adults, particularly men, do not like to admit that they are afraid. To be afraid means, in our society, that one is a coward. Actually, this is a false impression and, through her response of acceptance and respect, the nurse can demonstrate to the patient that it is natural for him to feel fear and that he should not view this as an affront to his self image.

How does the nurse demonstrate acceptance and respect? One effective means is through the response to questions asked. Patients may seem apologetic or embarrassed about some of the questions they have about their health or the treatment they are to receive. In the present day when there has been such a rapid change in educational systems and the expectations of everyone, people who have had fewer educational opportunities may feel embarrassed to know so little about their bodies. By offering direct and courteous answers, the nurse can convey the fact that questioning is quite appropriate and that no question is too small to deserve an answer. When questions arise that should be answered by the physician, the nurse has only to communicate this to the patient and then remind the patient to ask the physician when he visits the patient. A list of questions for the physician is a helpful reminder.

The matter of acceptance and respectful treatment is no more than practicing the common courtesies that should be a part of everyday living. The nurse should remember that to each patient his surgery is the most important surgery to be performed. Certainly, he is concerned about his neighbor, but no matter what happens, the self interest of the sick individual is primary. With this observation in mind, the nurse can accept each of her patients as individuals without resenting their individual demands.

The matter of spiritual care becomes very important to some pre-operative patients. Through her conversation with the patient as well as by familiarizing herself with his chart, the nurse can determine the wishes of the patient regarding a visit by his clergyman. People who are members of the Roman Catholic Church are usually visited by their priest prior to surgery. This practice is established sufficiently so that most nurses are aware of it. People of other faiths are frequently overlooked in this respect, however. The nurse should remember that many people of other faiths feel the need of the support which can be offered by their clergyman.

Other considerations pertaining to observation of the preoperative patient are more directly related to his physical preparation for surgery. The physical preparation can include several laboratory or other diagnostic studies, administration of intravenous fluids, blood transfusions, or demonstration and practice of exercises to be carried out after surgery. A urinalysis and complete blood count are almost always ordered to be done prior to surgery. Sometimes, additional studies may be ordered, such as hemoglobin and hematocrit levels. Also, such special studies as electrocardiogram, X-rays, or electroencephalogram may be done. And if it is anticipated that a patient will require blood transfusions at the time of surgery, there will be an order for blood to be typed and crossmatched. Policies vary as to whether the laboratory releases the blood to the operating room or to the patient's unit.

The nurse, knowing that these tests have been ordered, should be sure that their results have been returned and that the information is recorded properly on the chart. When the nurse reads the reports, she should look for any significant deviations from normal values so that the physician may be alerted. In some instances, he will deem remedy of the situation necessary prior to surgery. The importance of relieving any situations which may add to the risk of surgery cannot be under-estimated.

To evaluate the physical condition, the nurse should observe for the presence of any type of infection. An elevation in temperature may be an indication of infection and should be reported prior to sending patients to surgery. If a patient has a cough which is suggestive of pulmonary congestion, the nurse should report it. Many surgical procedures have been postponed because of the hazards of pulmonary congestion. The reason for this is that by the very requirement that the patient be kept quiet by means of anesthesia and sedation, his lungs will be less active. The tendency for fluid to accumulate in the lungs is increased by immobility which interferes with the normal excretion of mucus. The nurse should observe the general nutritional status of the patient by his weight and by the appearance of the skin. The loss of turgor may indicate that rapid weight loss has occurred, and this may be an indication for further study before surgery is attempted.

On the day of surgery, the nurse will measure and record the vital signs of the patient. The purpose of this is twofold. One purpose is to confirm the fitness of the patient to undergo surgery. Any deviation should be regarded seriously. The other purpose is to establish a norm with which the anesthetist, during surgery, and those caring for the patient after surgery can use for comparison with successive readings.

Cleanliness is another consideration in the preparation of the patient for surgery. The area immediately surrounding the site of the planned incision will be shaved and thoroughly cleaned with an antibacterial agent. The routine for surgical preparations varies in that some hospitals have technicians whose sole responsibility is to do the preoperative preparation of shaving and cleansing for all patients scheduled for surgery on the succeeding day. Other hospitals do not have such specialized categories of personnel, and the responsibility for the surgical preparation rests with the nurse on the unit. In either system, the nurse should examine the area prior to sending the patient to the operating room. While most of the preparations will be done well, the possibility of incorrect preparation does exist. Early detection of such a problem will save valuable time for the operating room staff.

The experience of a night nurse illustrates clearly how such a problem can arise and how steps can be taken to avert further difficulties. When the nurse was reviewing the orders pertaining to the care of a patient who was scheduled for surgical repair of a fractured right femur, she observed that the order had been written to prepare the appropriate area for repair of the left femur. Upon checking further, she discovered that, indeed, the left leg and hip area had been prepared. Fortunately, sufficient time remained to consult the physician for correction and to prepare the right leg. Although serious delay was averted, the patient was deprived of a good amount of rest during her preoperative night.

When assisting a patient with his daily hygiene prior to surgery, the nurse should observe for any evidence of bruises or any other types of injuries. The appearance of bruises may suggest that the patient has a tendency to bleed easily. If so, this should be known by the surgeon. Oral hygiene is an extremely important part of the preparation of a patient for surgery, too. The nurse should see to it that the patient either takes care of this himself or that he receives assistance with it. The importance of good oral hygiene lies in the removal of conditions which, when combined with the drying effects of medications used to reduce salivation during surgery, can contribute to the development of postoperative infections in the mouth.

Elimination from bowel and bladder is important for preoperative patients. Although the common practice for many years was to administer an enema prior to almost all types of surgery, many surgeons no longer include this in routine preparation. Situations which still would require this preparation would be those in which the abdominal viscera would be involved by the surgery. Otherwise, the main reason for emptying both bowel and bladder prior to surgery is the possibility of incontinence produced by the relaxant effects of anesthesia.

Sedatives are given at bedtime the night prior to surgery and again an hour or two before the patient leaves his room to insure his relaxation as the time for surgery approaches. The considerate nurse will see to it that a quiet environment is maintained throughout the period prior to surgery. Members of the family and the clergyman will be permitted to visit the patient prior to surgery, if desired. In all cases, the nurse should enlist their cooperation in providing a restful atmosphere by tactfully explaining to them exactly what is being done and the importance of rest. Rest is perhaps the most important part of the preparation of any patient for surgery.

The Operative Patient

When a patient arrives in the operating room suite or in one of its vestibules, he should be greeted by some member of the operating room nursing staff. All too often, he is left to lie on a stretcher for an indefinite period of time in a strange area filled with all sorts of peculiar sounds and odors without any greeting or reassurance from anyone. Even though the patient has received medication to help him relax, he still will respond to stimuli with confusion and worry. The nurse who receives the patient in the operating room should transport him to an area free from bright light and drafts. She should make sure that he has adequate covering to insure comfort, also.

Before anesthesia is administered, the patient should be reassured of his safety throughout the experience. This reassurance is provided best by the calm, yet concerned, manner in which both nurse and anesthetist treat the patient as an individual. During the time that a patient is undergoing surgery, the responsibility for observation of the patient rests with the anesthetist. Once the surgery has been completed, the patient will be taken to the recovery room where nurses will keep a constant watch over him until he regains consciousness and becomes aware of his surroundings. The anesthetist will supervise the care and progress of the patient throughout his stay in the recovery room. As soon as he deems it wise, he will authorize the nurse to return the patient to his room.

The Postoperative Patient

The sight of a patient who is recovering from anesthesia can be a rather startling one in that the patient may appear pale and lifeless. The process of recovery varies with the type of anethesia used, the type of surgery performed, the length of time the patient has been anesthetized, and his general condition before surgery.

During the immediate postoperative phase, there are some objectives of care which very directly involve nursing observations. They are: maintenance of an open airway, early detection of hemorrhage, early detection of shock, and maintenance of fluid and electrolyte balance. In order to maintain an open airway, the nurse must pay particular attention to the position of the patient, making sure at all times that his head is extended sufficiently to keep the nasopharynx free from obstruction. Also, an artificial airway may be inserted at the time of surgery and may be left in place until the patient is alert enough to push it out. Because of the medications administered prior to anesthesia, patients are less able to cough and expectorate the mucus that is secreted during the period of anesthesia. The nurse can tell if secretions are in the air passages by the noise made by air passing over them during respiration. Nasopharyngeal suctioning offers a means of removing the secretions until the patient is able to resume this function. The color, amount, and consistency of secretions removed should be noted.

The vital signs, i.e., blood pressure, pulse, and respirations, will be observed frequently during the immediate postoperative period. The blood pressure may fluctuate during this time as the pulse and respirations may do, also. One of the main objectives of postoperative care is to prevent the occurrence of shock. Although shock is not fully understood, it is known to occur as a result of severe trauma, blood loss, burns, surgery, pain, fear, infection, and as a reaction to some medications.

Shock represents an emergency situation, and quick action is required to restore adequate circulation. Observable characteristics of the patient in shock include drowsiness, apathetic expression, cold and clammy skin, cyanotic lips and nail beds, rapid and thready pulse, and shallow respirations. During the experience of shock, all of the body cells suffer from the lack of oxygen. Therefore, the entire physiological function of the body is impaired. Shock in the postoperative patient is not uncommon, and for this reason, the intravenous fluid therapy is continued until the blood pressure is stabilized. In the event that the patient should go into shock, the means to give fluids, blood, or medication would be established. It is very difficult to insert a needle into a vein that is collapsed.

When the nurse observes signs of impending shock, there are several things that she can do while awaiting the arrival of the physician. Some recovery rooms are equipped with beds that can be adjusted into the Trendelenburg position. If the beds cannot be operated this way, a straight chair placed under the foot of the bed will serve as a temporary arrangement. This can be done by one nurse if she places the chair, on its back, beneath the foot of the bed and pulls the top of the chair up to support the bed. As she continues to pull the chair upward and toward her, the foot of the bed will come to rest on the seat of the chair. The bed will roll a few inches toward the nurse, so caution should be exercised to protect any drainage bottles, tubing, or oxygen tanks. Additional blankets should be placed over the patient in shock to increase warmth. The emergency drug kit should be brought to the patient's unit so the physician will have whatever is needed.

As the nurse works with any postoperative patient, she should check the dressing over the incision periodically to ascertain whether there is bleeding. As the patient responds, his complaints of pain should be relieved by the administration of the medication ordered. Occasionally, sutures give way as a result of coughing or other stress on the incision. Complaints of pain and burning at the site of the incision should be respected and an examination made of the incision. When the sutures on an abdominal incision let go, it is possible for the contents of the abdomen to escape through this opening. This event is called evisceration. The nurse should cover the viscera quickly with sterile gauze which she has moistened with sterile saline solution. The patient will be taken back to surgery immediately for repair.

Patients who have had chest or abdominal surgery most likely will have drainage bottles which must be observed for the amount and characteristics of the contents. The bottles must be protected from breakage. The drainage bottles used to drain the wounds following chest surgery must be guarded most carefully because of the vacuum system which must be maintained. Breakage of the bottles or dislodging the tubing will permit air to enter the pleural space with a resultant pneumothorax. This complication could be very dangerous to the well-being of the patient.

As soon as the patient has recovered sufficiently from the anesthetic, he will be returned to his room where observation must continue, though it may not be by means of constant attendance. For safety's sake, the nurse should be sure that the patient who has just undergone surgery has siderails on his bed and that they are kept in position to protect him from rolling out of bed.

Explanations should be offered to the patient as soon as he is able to comprehend them, so that he understands the purpose of any soft restraints which have been applied to his arms for the protection of any tubes or bottles. Repeated reminders may be required as frequently as the patient awakens until he has recovered from the effects of the anesthesia and other medication. The depression of the central nervous system produced by these medications also causes the patient's level of awareness and span of memory to be impaired. Postoperative patients must not be expected to assume responsibility for watching their own intravenous fluids or for any other aspect of care for that matter.

As soon as the patient has recovered sufficiently from anesthesia, the nurse must see to it that he practices coughing and deep breathing to reexpand his lungs and prevent the development of infection. Fluid tends to collect in the lungs of a patient who lies quietly for an extended length of time and hypostatic pneumonia can develop. The nurse must assist the patient with deep coughing and breathing. Placing the hands over the incision will help to provide support as the patient coughs and may reduce the pain that the patient experiences upon coughing. It is not uncommon for patients to be afraid to cough, fearing that they will have severe pain or that they may cause injury to their incision. Changing position by turning from side to side helps to prevent pulmonary congestion also, and this should be done with regularity. Some patients develop respiratory complications in spite of preventive measures. When this happens, there are some observable symptoms. Some of them are: rapid respirations, fever, productive cough, copious amounts of sputum, difficulty in breathing, and chest pain. Because of her closer contact with the patient, it is frequently the nurse who first observes these symptoms.

Another problem in the care of many postoperative patients is that of mouth care. Prior to surgery, patients are given medication to reduce salivation, and depending upon the surgery performed, food and fluids by mouth may not be permitted for several hours or even days. During this time, the mouth becomes very dry and patients may complain of thirst. Ice chips afford welcome refreshment to patients who are so restricted. Maintenance of good mouth care by the nurse can help in the prevention of such complications as sordes and parotitis.

A rather common side effect of anesthetics is nausea and vomiting. Ether is especially noted for this undesirable effect. The problem exists until the gas is excreted. When a nurse observes a patient who is nauseated, she should help him to maintain a position which will enable him to get rid of the vomitus. Aspiration of such liquids can be a hazard to respiratory function. The amount, color, and consistency of any vomitus should be observed and recorded. In some instances, nausea may cause retching without vomiting. When this happens, it can cause much discomfort to the patient. Persistent nausea should be called to the attention of the physician.

Postoperative patients often complain of a backache. This is caused by remaining in the same position on the flat surface of the operating table. Change of position and a backrub with particular attention to the small of the back will help to relieve this discomfort.

It is essential that the nurse observe the amount and characteristics of urinary output following surgery. The effects of the anesthesia along with the lower intake of food and fluids cause some patients to have difficulty voiding after surgery. The medication causes a loss in muscle tone of the bladder, and urination is thereby suppressed. Sometimes, such suggestive measures as running water within hearing distance, pouring warm water over the vulva of the female, or placing the hands in warm water may be of value in assisting the patient to void. If all of these measures fail, catheterization may be the only alternative. The nurse can detect a distended urinary bladder by gently palpating the area just above the symphysis pubis where it can be palpated as a firm, round mass.

Some additional complications that can occur following surgery are thrombophlebitis, pulmonary embolism, wound infection, and perito-nitis. Whenever the postoperative patient is observed to have an ele-vated temperature, the possibility of any of these complications should be considered. When a patient develops thrombophlebitis as a result of the stasis brought about by inactivity, the nurse probably will be able to observe redness and swelling of the lower leg. Also, the patient may complain of pain in the calf of his leg. If the patient has been ambulatory, the nurse should ask him to remain in bed until the phy-sician can examine his leg. It is best to avoid frightening the patient by suggesting development of complications, but the nurse should know that, in the presence of thrombophlebitis, massage or exercise could cause a clot to break away and to move along to the lung where it would become a pulmonary embolism.

Pulmonary embolism is characterized by severe chest pain which may be accompanied by bloody sputum. The patient may appear to be in shock as a result of the pain. Pulmonary embolism is a potentially dangerous complication because of the possibility of obstruction of the pulmonary artery. Such an obstruction could be fatal.

Although much attention has been focused upon the study of prevention and control of wound infections, they still pose serious problems which can prolong the hospital stay of the patient.[2] For a breadwinner, such an experience could have disastrous effects. When the nurse changes the dressing covering the incision, she should pay particular attention to the condition of the wound. Redness, swelling, and purulent drainage are signs which should be reported.

While improved surgical techniques and antibiotic therapy have reduced the incidence of peritonitis, it is still important for the nurse to be aware of the symptoms of it. Patients who have had intestinal surgery are particularly susceptible to this problem. The occurrence of a high temperature, abdominal distention, and intense pain may signal this complication. Immediate treatment is necessary to control and relieve this problem.

Severity and duration of pain experienced by postoperative patients will vary with the type of surgery performed. In addition to administering the prescribed analgesic, the nurse must evaluate its effectiveness. Persistent pain should be reported to the physician. Generally, the need for medication to relieve pain diminishes as healing occurs. Detailed discussion of observation of the patient with pain can be found in Chapter 3.

It should be remembered that the experience of surgery and all of its discomforts can produce mild, temporary behavioral changes in people. The tendency to become self-centered at the time of surgery is a perfectly natural one, and as the patient regains his strength, he can be expected to resume his usual characteristics. The fears of the postoperative patient can be just as important and prevalent as those of the preoperative patient. Characteristically, people have been made

---

[2]Shirley Streeter, Helen Dunn, and Mark Lepper, "Hospital Infections — A Necessary Risk?" *American Journal of Nursing*, Vol. 67, No. 3, 1967, page 526.

to feel that they relinquish all rights when they enter the hospital.[3] Leaders in the nursing profession today are working diligently to improve the quality of nursing care by making it more individualized. The sensitive nurse will acknowledge the rights of patients to ask ques· tions and to understand what is happening to them.

A good illustration can be observed in the case of a man who, at the age of fifty-four, underwent heart surgery. On one occasion when the surgeon visited the patient, there was discussion about plans to remove the tube which led from the chest to the drainage bottles. The patient listened unquestioningly. As the nurse worked with him later, however, the patient asked what would happen to his chest when the tube would be removed. Realizing his concern, the nurse explained what was to be done and then asked what had caused the patient to ask this question. The patient admitted to fears that removal of the tube would leave a large defect in his chest wall through which air could pass. He knew that air rushing into the chest cavity could produce harmful and possibly even fatal results to him. Obtaining explicit information helped him to relax. Not all questions pertain to such vital problems, but as soon as the patient expresses the need for information, explanations should be offered.

When patients are permitted out of bed following surgery, the nurse should stay with them until she is sure they are strong enough to manage alone. The usual process is to permit the patient to sit on the side of the bed with his feet down for a short while to see how well he can tolerate the change in position. If no untoward effects occur, the patient can be assisted out of bed. It must be remembered that patients who have been lying flat for any length of time are quite likely to experience dizziness upon assuming the upright position. Patients who have undergone surgery will be weak and should be provided assistance until the nurse is sure of the patient's ability to tolerate activity.

Postoperative care of many patients continues beyond discharge from the hospital. Because of the early ambulation and shortened hospital stay, most patients are required to return either to the outpatient clinic or to the physician's office for follow-up care. Nurses should never assume that patients just know what care they should have but, instead, should develop a plan of instructions to be given before the patient leaves the hospital. Instructions should be started as soon as the patient is able to accept them. Allowing the patient to participate in his care is a very important part of this teaching. As he learns of his

---

[3]Carol Dickinson Taylor, "Sociological Sheep Shearing," *Nursing Forum*, Vol. 1, No. 2, 1962, page 80.

limitations and ways to manage them, fears of discharge from the hospital will be alleviated.

THE PATIENT DURING A SEIZURE

There are many situations in which the nurse is called upon to describe a seizure which has been experienced by a patient. It is the nurse who is most likely to be present, since the occurrence of such episodes is highly unpredictable. Seizures occur with many kinds of medical problems ranging from anxiety reactions to serious cerebral pathology. An anxious or a very weak person may experience a seizure as a result of hyperventilation. For example, a patient who has had surgery and is beginning to ambulate probably will feel very weak. Some people have a tendency to begin deep breathing in such situations of stress, and their respirations are characterized by longer expiratory phases than inspiratory phases. As a result, an excessive amount of carbon dioxide is excreted, and the physiologic response may be a generalized seizure. This is brought about by the interference with the respiratory center and the supply of oxygen to the brain.

Seizures which occur as a result of brain pathology may or may not have rather characteristic patterns. At first, the patient may experience an aura or a period when he is aware that something is wrong, but he is unable to do anything about it. There may be such symptoms as a cry, muscle twitching, or a change in facial expression. When the seizure is accompanied by an aura, the nurse must be alert to the signs of its development so that she can take the necessary measures to insure the safety of the patient as the seizure progresses. When the nurse or patient recognizes the onset of this phase, the patient should be assisted into bed so that physical injury resulting from falling can be prevented.

As the seizure progresses, the nurse should observe the exact parts of the body that are involved in the twitching or severe contractions that follow. She should take note of the length of each phase. The length of the seizure may seem to be much longer than it actually is because of its frightening aspects. During the convulsive phase, the nurse must position the patient's head in such a way that his tongue does not obstruct his breathing. Padded tongue blades are a necessity at the bedside of any patient who is susceptible to seizures. Their purpose is to maintain an open airway during the convulsive phase. They must be inserted before the convulsion begins, however.

At the end of the convulsive phase, the patient will relax, and he may regain consciousness immediately with only some slight confusion as to his whereabouts or he may lapse into a deep sleep which may last for several minutes. All of these aspects should be observed closely so that a complete descriptive account can be provided the physician. A record of all seizures that occur is essential in determining a pattern of occurrence and involvement.

Regardless of the cause of a seizure, the nurse must be aware of its danger to the patient. Application of padded side rails to the patient's bed will help to prevent injury from falling out of bed or from bumping the hard metal.

Children are subject to seizures when marked elevations in temperature occur. This can happen as children encounter the various diseases common to childhood or the numerous respiratory infections that can occur. Children should be protected with the same precautions as adults, and in addition, parents should be instructed in the care of their children during this episode. When parents are taught how to protect their children, they can perform in an effective way rather than being rendered helpless by fear.

THE TERMINALLY ILL PATIENT

Nursing care of the terminally ill patient is a challenging task for any nurse. It is always the hope of those who are responsible for the patient's care that life can be prolonged. Even when the situation appears to be without hope, nurses and physicians do what they can to promote life with the hope of finding some way to reduce the suffering of the patient.

As the nurse works with patients who are so critically ill, much of her care will be directed toward providing as much comfort as she can for the patient. While the debate about the use of extraordinary measures to preserve life continues, the task of the nurse is still to offer as much help as she can. The meaning of death to the patient is a consideration which is often overlooked. The nurse should attempt to understand the fears being experienced by the patient as he sees himself growing weaker and closer to death.[4]

Many of the observations that will be made as life ebbs will be related to the failing circulatory system. The hands, feet, ears, and nose will become pale and cold. The nails will take on the bluish discoloration which is typical of cyanosis. There may be excessive per-

---

[4]C. Knight Aldrich, "The Dying Patient's Grief," *Journal of the American Medical Association,* 177:1963, pages 329-31; Barney G. Glaser and Anselm L. Strauss, "The Social Loss of Dying Patients," *American Journal of Nursing,* Vol. 64, No. 6, 1964, page 119.

spiration as the skin takes on a pale or perhaps a mottled appearance. The pulse will become weaker and may not even be palpable over the radial artery. The blood pressure will fall and eventually will be inaudible.

The respirations of the dying patient may change in character, becoming slower and more shallow. Sometimes Cheyne Stokes respirations occur with intermittent periods of very rapid breathing which fades away to periods of apnea or no breathing. Sometimes, noise can be heard with respirations. This noise is caused by air passing over the collections of mucus in the throat. These secretions accumulate because of the patient's inability to cough or expectorate.

The muscles gradually lose tone so that the patient lies rather limply in whatever position he happens to be placed. The jaw may sag, and speech becomes difficult for the patient and difficult for the nurse to understand. The eyes become sunken and partially closed. Reflexes disappear, including the reaction of pupils to light. In fact, the failure of the pupils to respond to light is one of the most conclusive signs of impending death.

The attitude of dying patients varies. Some patients will appear to be frightened and restless while others seem to relax and move gradually into a deeper sleep until life ceases. The sense of hearing is believed to be one of the last senses to cease functioning, and for this reason, the room should be kept quiet and caution exercised in conversations among hospital personnel.

The death of some people comes about very suddenly, and there is no opportunity to observe these signs. When a sudden death occurs, the nurse should move quietly and quickly to summon assistance. Then, her attention should be directed toward the supportive care of any patients who are nearby and who may be aware of what has transpired. The occurrence of death cannot be a secret to all patients. While some will be unsuspecting, others will realize what has happened and the nurse must be honest with them. There is no need for the nurse to go into details about what has happened, but other patients, who are aware of the death, must be permitted to release their feelings. Otherwise, the anxiety that festers can only produce mental anguish which can be detrimental.

During all of this very emotionally charged time, the family of the patient must not be forgotten. For the support of one another, families need to be together. Nurses can be helpful to families if they will only show them the consideration needed. Relatives should be encouraged to maintain their own health and should be provided directions to facilities where food and rest can be obtained. Some cultures require that all members of the family be present throughout the last days of the life of one of its members. The desire to uphold these traditions sometimes is carried over into the American culture, but since most hospitals are not built to accommodate large numbers of relatives at any one time, other arrangements must be made. Great patience is required of the nurse in working with groups like this so that she can provide understanding assistance.

The nurse must be alert, too, to the effects of such stress and shock as death presents and may have to assist any relatives who are unable to tolerate this experience. A supply of spirits of ammonia is an essential in any ward situation. In the event that a relative does become faint or extremely emotional, medical assistance should be sought.

In the crucial time as death approaches, the patient or his family may desire the presence of his clergyman, and it may be the nurse who must summon him. The presence of the clergyman may offer immeasurable support to the family in this time of crisis. Some patients may find it difficult to request the nurse to call a clergyman, and it is quite appropriate for the nurse to take the initiative in offering the suggestion. When patients come from a distance, they may be unfamiliar with the clergymen in the area in which the hospital is located. Many hospitals have chaplain service either on a full-time or part-time basis. When there is a chaplain available, his services can be requested to help with such emergencies. However, the clergyman can offer much more understanding assistance if he has been seeing a patient and his family throughout the period of illness. In no case should everyone wait until the patient is dying to seek the services of his clergyman.

While many books have been written about death and its impact upon the family, one that is suggested reading is, *Death Be Not Proud*.[5] The student of nursing will do well to read some of this literature and to think about it to help her work through her own feelings and attitudes regarding death. Only when she has resolved some of her own feelings about death will she be able to function calmly in its wake and to recognize the needs of all concerned.

THE GERIATRIC PATIENT

Although population experts predict that by 1970 one-half of the population of this country will be under the age of twenty-five, there is still a growing number of people in the aging population group, and if current trends continue, one can anticipate even greater life ex-

---

[5]John Gunther, *Death Be Not Proud* (New York: Harper and Brothers, 1949).

pectancy in the years to come. As the span of life has increased even in this century, the problems of the medical care of the aged have mushroomed. The cost of medical care and hospitalization exceeds by far the ability of the average retired person to pay. Retirement benefits which were planned some thirty or forty years ago cannot rise proportionately with the rises in the cost of living. Therefore, the problem of maintaining oneself without the extra expense of hospitalization and medications sometimes seems almost prohibitive. Then when illness strikes, it poses an impossible burden.

The nurse will meet many of these elderly persons through her experiences in the hospital. It is difficult for the young person of twenty to twenty-five to understand the real nature of the problems of adjustment to old age. To the young, old age seems so remote that it hardly seems worth thinking about. But the young nurse must learn about the problems of aging if she is to develop understanding of the fears and problems confronting the aged person. Because of the emphasis upon youth in the American society, the very thoughts of growing old are disturbing.

What are some of the observations, then, of the aged patient? First, perhaps it should be said that to identify any specific age as the division between middle age and old age is impossible. Some people will seem younger at eighty than others will seem at sixty. Suffice it to say that there are observable physiologic and psychologic changes that occur with aging that require consideration.

One of the first changes that can be observed is the condition of the skin. The skin of the elderly patient appears dry and transparent because of the loss of subcutaneous fat. The skin loses its turgor, and wrinkles are prevalent. The skin actually becomes thinner and is more fragile causing it to be more prone to injury. Healing of injuries occurs more slowly because of the general decline of cell metabolism. The appendages, the hair, and the nails change too. The hair becomes more difficult to manage and may become thinner, even in women. Some women develop problems with the appearance of coarse, facial hairs. Regardless of her age, a woman likes to be as attractive as possible, and all of these changes are disturbing to elderly women who see themselves gradually degenerating.

Another area of change is in the musculoskeletal system. The fact that these people are less steady on their feet increases their chances of falling, and the decrease in the adequacy of calcium metabolism causes the bones to be more brittle. Hence, there is a relatively high incidence of fractures among elderly people. Because of the general decrease in muscle strength, the maintenance of good support is essential whether these people are sitting in a chair or lying in bed. The soft, overstuffed chair is no place for the elderly patient. The flexibility required to get into and out of the chair makes it inconvenient if not uncomfortable. The elderly patient finds it difficult to manipulate his stiff joints with any degree of haste, and for this reason, plenty of time should be allowed for movement.

Due to the wear and tear through years of use, the joints in the hands may be quite large and stiff. The type of arthritis that occurs as a part of the degenerative process is not as crippling as the more acute arthritis, but even so, marked deformities of the hands and fingers can result. Because of the joint stiffness and pain, fine movements become difficult.

As efficiency of the circulatory system decreases, the patient becomes chilled more easily. A warm hot water bottle or electric blanket can be used to provide warmth as he sleeps. Heating pads are of some value, but there is more danger of burning with the heating pad because of the intense and continuous heat produced.

Changes occur in the condition of the blood vessels as well as in the efficiency of the heart. With the gradual process of hardening, or arteriosclerosis, the vessels lose their elasticity causing a greater resistance to the circulating blood. The result is that the heart must work harder to accomplish its purpose. This in turn increases the strain upon heart muscle which is suffering the effects of continuous labor throughout the many years. The increased resistance in the arterial walls can cause an increase in the blood pressure which adds to the work of the heart. The cycle becomes more vicious, and the patient becomes more prone to circulatory problems.

With all of these degenerative changes in circulation, the patient becomes a more likely candidate for the dreaded and debilitating problem of cerebral vascular accidents commonly known as strokes. This problem can be caused either by hemorrhage or obstruction of cerebral vessels by some type of thrombus or embolus. In either case, the patient is apt to suffer paralysis of the entire part of his body which is controlled by the involved portion of the brain. He may lose the ability to speak as well as his control over elimination. All of these problems are very depressing to the elderly patient, and the nursing care directed toward rehabilitation is extremely challenging. People who have suffered the circulatory changes that accompany arteriosclerosis often cry easily, and the nurse working with them must understand this problem so that she can continue to show the kindness and consideration that is needed so desperately.

As the aging patient loses his ability to control elimination, the problems of urinary frequency, dribbling, or retention occur. In the presence of dribbling, the odor becomes difficult to control. The elderly patient is bothered greatly by his loss of independence in the care of these functions. Therefore, assistance given should be offered in a straightforward manner which calls as little attention to the disability as possible.

Nutritional problems of the elderly patient increase as loss of appetite occurs with less expenditure of physical energy. Not only are they less interested in food, but the ability to digest foods is impaired by the degenerative changes occurring in the gastrointestinal tract. Small feedings of bland but nutritious foods should be offered as frequently as the patient can tolerate them. Effort should be exerted to serve foods that are attractive and appetizing.

With less strenuous physical activity, less demand is placed upon the respiratory organs. Resulting respiratory changes cause the elderly patient to be more susceptible to infections. For this reason, they should protect themselves or should be protected from exposure to other people who have infections.

The senses of sight, hearing, smell, taste, and touch become impaired with progressive degenerative changes. Attention should be given to failing eyes so that vision is retained as long as possible. Magnifying glasses can be very helpful to the person with poor vision. The use of hearing aids may seem annoying and cumbersome at first, but once the adjustment has been made, the person with impaired hearing will derive much pleasure from being able to participate in conversations rather than feeling outside the group because he cannot hear what is being said. Those who converse with him should remember to speak clearly and distinctly in natural tones. The lower tones can be heard much better than the higher tones which are likely to be utilized in shouting.

The incidence of diabetes increases in the aging population as does the susceptibility to various other degenerative disorders. For this reason, any aged person should have periodic physical examinations to facilitate early detection and treatment of medical problems.

With all of these physical changes occurring, another change occurs which is not the least of the problems in the care of the aging population. The psychologic impact of retirement and the facing of old age causes many people to feel that they have reached an age of uselessness. They have seen their children mature and assume the responsibility of families of their own. When society was less mobile, the proximity of living facilities was much greater. In the present age, with the approaching realization of space travel, families become much more widely scattered. Realizing that such changes do occur, the time to begin preparing for the so-called "golden years" is during a much earlier period in life. The development of hobbies and varied interests is essential for the aged person to find ways to fill the time that hangs so heavily when all routines have ceased. It is important that the aged person remain active as long as he is able. He should try to seek the company of others who have similar interests as the support offered by people with common problems and interests is immeasurable.

Finding help to care for the aging invalid at home or making other suitable arrangements becomes a difficult problem as the aged patient approaches the stage at which constant hospital care is no longer needed. Many of these patients will be depressed because they have no one who can take care of them, or as they see it, no one to care. Fortunately, the rising social concern in this country is offering hope for many. Through the personal efforts of the nurse in the hospital and community, these people can be guided to a richer, fuller life.

SUMMARY

While it is recognized that every patient is an individual, the situations presented in this chapter provide examples of application of the knowledge of observation to the care of the specific patient. Whether the patient is observed in the hospital, in the outpatient clinic, or in the home, the nurse must keep in mind the meaning of illness to the patient and should administer to his needs accordingly.

BIBLIOGRAPHY

ALDRICH, C. KNIGHT, "The Dying Patient's Grief," *Journal of the American Medical Association*, 177:1963, p. 329-31.

BELAND, IRENE L., *Clinical Nursing*. New York: The Macmillan Company, 1965.

CARNEVALI, DORIS, "Preoperative Anxiety," *American Journal of Nursing*, Vol. 66, No. 7, 1966, p. 1536-1538.

COULTER, PEARL PARVIN, *The Nurse in the Public Health Program*. New York: G. P. Putnam's Sons, 1954.

ENGLAND, RICHEL H., "Public Health Nursing In Child Care Homes," *American Journal of Nursing*, Vol. 67, No. 1, 1967, p. 114-116.

FREEMAN, RUTH B., *Public Health Nursing Practice*. Philadelphia: W. B. Saunders Company, 1957.

GLASER, BARNEY G., and STRAUSS, ANSELM L., "The Social Loss of Dying Patients," *American Journal of Nursing*, Vol. 64, No. 6, 1964, p. 119.

GUNTHER, JOHN, *Death Be Not Proud.* New York: Harper and Brothers, Publishers, 1949.

KAUTZ, HAROLD D., *et. al.,* "Radioactive Drugs," *American Journal of Nursing,* Vol. 64, No. 1, 1964, p. 24.

LIEBEN, JAN, "The Effects of Radiation," *Nursing Outlook,* Vol. 10, No. 5, 1962, p. 336-338.

MATHENEY, RUTH V., and others, *Fundamentals of Patient-Centered Nursing.* St. Louis: The C. V. Mosby Company, 1964.

NOLES, EVA M., "Nursing A Geriatric Patient," *American Journal of Nursing,* Vol. 63, No. 1, 1963, p. 73-74.

PIRNIE, FLORENCE, and BALDWIN, MARTLAND, "Observing Cerebral Seizures," *American Journal of Nursing,* Vol. 59, No. 3, 1959, p. 366-369.

QUINT, JEANNE C., "Obstacles to Helping the Dying," *American Journal of Nursing,* Vol. 66, No. 7, 1966, p. 1568-1571.

RODSTEIN, MANUEL, "The Aging Process and Disease," *Nursing Outlook,* Vol. 12, No. 11, 1964, p. 43.

SKAGGS, LESTER, and HAUGHEY, ROSEMARY, "Radioactive Isotope Therapy," *Nursing Outlook,* Vol. 6, No. 4, 1958, p. 214-216.

SMITH, DOROTHY W., and GIPS, CLAUDIA D., *Care of the Adult Patient,* 2nd ed. Philadelphia: J. B. Lippincott Company, 1966.

STAFFORD, NOVA HARRIS, "Bowel Hygiene of Aged Patients," *American Journal of Nursing,* Vol. 63, No. 9, 1963, p. 102.

STREETER, SHIRLEY, DUNN, HELEN, and LEPPER, MARK, "Hospital Infections — A Necessary Risk?" *American Journal of Nursing,* Vol. 67, No. 3, 1967, p. 526-533.

TAYLOR, CAROL DICKINSON, "Sociological Sheep Shearing," *Nursing Forum,* Vol. 1, No. 2, 1962, p. 80.

WIEDENBACH, ERNESTINE, "The Helping Art of Nursing," *American Journal of Nursing,* Vol. 63, No. 11, 1963, p. 54.

WESTBERG, GRANGER, *Nurse, Pastor and Patient.* Rock Island, Illinois: Augustana Press, 1955.

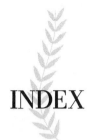

INDEX